Ward Sister at Work

With good wishes.
from

[signature]

February 95

STUDIES IN NURSING SERIES

Already published

Psychiatric Nursing Described
Desmond F.S. Cormack

Learning to Nurse — Integrating Theory and Practice
Margaret F. Alexander

Forthcoming title

Postnatal Care — The Midwives' Role
Maureen Laryea

Ward Sister at Work

Phyllis J. Runciman
BSc MPhil RGN SCM HV Cert
Research Associate, Nursing Research
Unit, University of Edinburgh

Foreword by
Pat Ashworth
MSc SRN SCM FRCN
Research Programme Manager, WHO
Collaborating Centre, Department
of Nursing, University of Manchester

CHURCHILL LIVINGSTONE
EDINBURGH LONDON MELBOURNE AND NEW YORK 1983

CHURCHILL LIVINGSTONE
Medical Division of Longman Group Limited

Distributed in the United States of America by
Churchill Livingstone Inc., 1560 Broadway, New York,
N.Y. 10036, and by associated companies, branches and
representatives throughout the world.

Longman Group Limited 1983

First published 1983

ISBN 0 443 02622 X

British Library Cataloguing in Publication Data
Runciman, Phyllis
    Ward sister at work. — (Studies in nursing)
    1. Nursing service administration — Great Britain
    2. Nurse administrators — Great Britain
    I. Title   II. Series
    362.1'1'068   RT89

Library of Congress Cataloging in Publication Data
Runciman, Phyllis J.
    Ward sister at work.
    (Studies in nursing series)
    Bibliography: p.
    Includes index.
    1. Nursing — Social aspects. 2. Nurses —
    Attitudes.
3. Nurses — Scotland — Interviews. I. Title. II.
Series.
[DNLM: 1. Nursing — Scotland. 2. Nursing,
Supervisory.
WY 105 R939w]
RT86.5.R86   1983   610.73'06'9   82–17794

Printed in Singapore by Huntsmen Offset Printing Pte Ltd

Foreword

Many patients, nurses, students, doctors and others have in past years regarded the ward sister as a most important factor in the general atmosphere, morale, efficiency and effectiveness of any hospital ward. Despite the 'dragon' image of some, sisters have been rewarded with the respect and sometimes gratitude and affection of these people, even if not with high salaries. Increasingly one hears of patients who 'hardly see Sister' or are not sure if there is one. Students sometimes make similar complaints.

There have been many changes over the last 25 years — shorter working hours, more part-time staff, more and older patients staying shorter times in hospital, more technology, centralisation of some services, reorganisation of others, industrial relations problems, more demands from the nursing school for student objectives and assessments. All these and many other factors affect ward sisters in their attempt to fulfil their own and others' expectations of a ward sister. Despite the changes and problems, some ward sisters seem to cope well, sometimes for a number of years. But at what personal cost? Why do some survive better than others? Why do others behave in ways which are less helpful to those for whom they have responsibility, such as patients and their relatives, and nursing students?

There have been several studies of the ward sister's performance — as manager (Pembrey 1980), as leader and in relation to students and the learning environment (Fretwell 1980, Orton 1981, Ogier 1982) and job satisfaction (Redfern 1981). Much of the essential activity of the ward sister is not visible, it goes on in her head. It may well be perceptions, thinking process and feelings which are important in the provision of an optimal 'climate' for recovery, for nursing and other health care, and for learning, as much as external resources and circumstances; although obviously each may influence the others. Phyllis Runciman has produced a study which gives insight into the world of 'sistering' as perceived by nine ward sisters, their descriptions and comments on problems being linked with more structured measures and observational data. Her critical yet sympathetic interpretations of the data and indeed the whole study are grounded in her own experience of a love–hate relationship with the job of a ward sister.

There is much talk of stress in nursing at present, and with all the complex and demanding aspects of her job a ward sister seems to be subject to the kind of pressures which may produce negative reactions to stress. Yet increasingly it is being recognised that the same kinds of things may produce satisfaction or negative reaction to stress. It depends on the individuals' perceptions of the situation and their ability to use coping mechanisms which produce benefit for themselves and others. For example, some of the sisters in this study wanted more staff, yet also perceived it as a problem when there was staff but little perceived work. As the author says, some of them convey a disturbing impression of fatalism and a feeling of powerlessness to do anything about their problems. This is a poor basis from which to provide management, leadership and teaching.

Perhaps the answer is to give time and help to both individuals and groups of ward sisters to think through the problems they face, to decide what aspects can be changed and ways of doing so, and to identify strategies and coping methods which can be used deliberately when circumstances cannot be changed. Those who have lost their sense of purpose and control in the fragmentation and complexity of their activities may then regain it. This study provides an excellent basis for such endeavours. May success attend the author and others who use it to help ward sisters (those who need help) to be people who 'accept the role of pilot rather than of robot' (Knowles & Saxberg 1971), who initiate, plan and control rather than just react, and who enjoy what can be one of the most satisfying as well as valuable jobs that exist.

Manchester 1983   Pat Ashworth

Details of references are on page 127.

Preface

'So you want to know about the heaven and the hell of sistering.' That was the response of one sister* when asked if she would like to talk about her work and its problems and to participate in the research upon which this book is based. The research study was carried out in 1976 and 1977 with a small sample of nine sisters from medical and surgical wards in two district general hospitals in Scotland. Its aim was to identify problems experienced by ward sisters and to explore in depth, using a case-study approach, the sisters' own views about day-to-day work difficulties.

The author's special interest in this topic arose from personal experience as a medical ward sister for three years immediately before the study. The experience was challenging and enjoyable. It was also endlessly frustrating and created the kind of love–hate relationship with the job that seemed to be shared by the sister who made the opening remark above.

The work of the sister is extremely varied and the physical and emotional demands of the job can be heavy. As the nine sisters in this study describe their experiences, they bring to life the untidy reality of their daily work and its problems. Some of their remarks are perceptive, amusing and thought-provoking. But many comments are disturbing, and reinforce the current concern in the profession about the state of development of this important nursing role.

This book is therefore for all who are interested in the work of the ward sister. In particular, it is for sisters themselves and for their manager and teacher colleagues, who should be working together to improve not only the preparation for the job but also the day-to-day support and continuing education which such complex work demands.

Edinburgh 1983   P.J.R.

---

* For convenience, the term 'sister' and the feminine gender are used throughout to include both ward sisters and charge nurses.

Acknowledgements

I am grateful to the Scottish Home and Health Department for the award of a nursing research training fellowship, which made possible the study of ward sisters upon which this book is based.

During the two years of the fellowship, many members of staff and students of the Nursing Research Unit and the Department of Nursing Studies of the University of Edinburgh gave me their enthusiastic support and their constructive criticism. I am grateful to them and to Dr Lisbeth Hockey and Professor Annie Altschul for their instruction and encouragement.

I should like to express my thanks to the Health Boards in Scotland and to the many nurse management teams for their cooperation throughout the study, and my profound thanks go to all the sisters who welcomed me to their wards and gave me so much of their valuable time. I greatly appreciated their courteous hospitality and the very thoughtful consideration which they gave to this research.

Finally my special thanks go to the sisters and their colleagues in management and education whose interest in the findings of the research encouraged me to write this book.

P.J.R.

Contents

1

Sister and her work

What are 'occult messages' and when are they a problem? Why do sisters worry about being too busy and dislike being too quiet? What is wrong with the traditional system of learning the sister's job? Why is there conflict between sisters and doctors and tension between sisters and nursing officers?

Answers to these and other questions about the work of ward sisters will be given by the nine in this study as they talk about their day-to-day worries and problems. To set the scene to their problems, this chapter looks back to long-established traditions in nursing and to some recent changes in the health professions and in society which have shaped the work of today's sisters.

The ward sister is often described as the key figure, or linchpin, in the organisation of a ward and in the management of patient care. Since the 1970s the spotlight has been turned increasingly on the complex nature of the administrative, clinical and teaching responsibilities of the role and it has been recognised that acting as coordinator at the centre of a wide network of people, services and communications is a complicated and demanding job. Many aspects of ward work have become the subject of debate and research, and studies have shown that some of the most valuable skills used by sisters are urgently in need of development; for example, skills in communication, in teaching and in management (Lelean 1973, Bendall 1976, Pembrey 1980). Concern about the sister was summed up by McFarlane (1976) in her remark that the sister's role, which had been 'developed for a very different era', had become inefficient and had failed to adapt to change.

PAST TRADITION

The influence of the past is still evident in the work of today's sisters; for example, in their close working relationships with doctors, in their styles of leadership within the nursing team and in their role as teachers in the apprenticeship system of nurse training.

1

Trained nurse and teacher

In the early 1800s nursing was considered a menial job for the un-educated. By the turn of the nineteenth century it was becoming acceptable as a suitable career for women, and the idea was de-veloping that a trained professional nurse of good character should be able to understand the nature of her patients' conditions and in-telligently assist the doctor.

Sisters in Florence Nightingale's time were selected from lady pupils rather than from the probationers. They paid for one year of training and having gained a certificate many were sent throughout Britain taking with them principles of training from St Thomas' Hospital, London, one such principle being that the practical teaching of nurses should be carried out in the ward under the direction of the sister. After a century of debate and change in the form of nurse education and the development of classroom-based instruction, the Royal Commission on the National Health Service reaffirmed in 1979 that 'clinical practice is the "core" of nursing education; clinical practice is best taught by practising nurses in real situations' (p. 202).

Today, sisters can no longer be so clearly distinguished from other nurses by social class, age and education. The sister is no longer the 'lady' in the midst of servant classes. She is not necessarily older or better educated; in fact, she may be considerably younger than some nurses in her team. Also, with changes in educational entry to nursing and with the development of college and university based nursing courses, it has been suggested that some sisters now perceive themselves as less well-educated than the learners whom they instruct and supervise (Mackenzie 1973).

Sister and doctor

The nature of the relationship between nurse and doctor has also changed during the past century, from that of handmaiden to part-ner. In the early 1800s sisters acted mainly as domestic supervisors and their principal responsibility was to see that doctors' orders were carried out. They were also taught by doctors, and Abel-Smith (1960) tells us that in 1830 in St Bartholomew's Hospital, London, sisters were reported to have 'an admirable sagacity and a sort of rough practical knowledge which was nearly as good as any acquired skill' (p. 9).

Doctors also played a major role in appointments and dismissals of sisters. In the records of rules and regulations for the Lady Super-intendent of Nurses in the Royal Infirmary of Edinburgh, dur-ing 1881 it is reported (p. 22): 'No Head Nurse shall be dismissed without the circumstances of the case having been previously referred to the Physician or Surgeon to whose ward she is attached.' In the same hospital the minutes of a nursing committee over 40 years later recorded in 1925 that the committee acceded to the request of two physician heads of departments that their respective ward sisters be retained beyond their planned retiral age for a further period of one to two years until the physicians themselves retired. Unfortunately no reasons are given for this apparent accolade, and one is left wondering whether it arose from an appreciation of the skill and 'admirable sagacity' of those sisters, from a wish to extend an impecunious spinster's useful earning life or simply from a reluctance to have to adapt to a new sister's ways.

Today, a sister is expected to be able to think and act independently on nursing matters. She needs to be aware of the complementary nature of nurse–doctor roles and of the interdependence of members of a ward team in decision-making. However, despite talk of partnership, tensions still exist at the boundaries between medicine and nursing (British Medical Journal 1981).

It often seems that shared dialogue and harmony between sister and doctor is still more myth than reality. Some sisters lack confidence. They feel threatened by doctors and are reluctant to express their opinions on nursing matters. Some doctors fail to consider the nursing viewpoint and to acknowledge the importance of the nurse's contribution to patient care. Traditional, outdated attitudes persist in the 1980s and such attitudes can hinder professional development.

'Dragons' and discipline

The lingering authoritarianism in nursing also has its roots in the past.

The image is still real of the 'old battleaxe' ward sister, the feared but respected disciplinarian who was found, surprisingly, to have a heart of gold despite asperity of tongue and unapproachable manner. Authoritarian management helped to maintain efficiency and possibly provided some security for patients, nurses and sisters, but it undoubtedly stifled progress and was restrictive, petty and inhuman.

Independence of thought, freedom to question and speak out were discouraged among probationer nurses and such traditions die hard. The legacy of the 'dragon' sister and the inhibited student nurse remains. MacGuire (1961) and Revans (1964) found that student nurses regarded some sisters as uncommunicative and unapproachable; poor communication was thought to restrict teaching and to reduce the likelihood of the sister being seen as a source of help and information. A decade later, Anderson (1973) was given the response 'Petty sisters with petty rules' in answer to questions about current problems in nursing.

Restrictive rules and limited communication also influence relationships between sister and patients. Most of the few criticisms of sisters by patients in Cartwright's (1964) study concerned authoritarian attitudes. Cartwright did point out, however, that while some patients described the sister as strict, others felt that she was not strict enough; when she was too lenient with the nurses, the patients suffered.

The tradition of a disciplined approach to work has also contributed to the strict adherence to routine which is so often found in nursing.

Routinisation of some aspects of work can be sensible and helpful. Nevertheless it has been found that adhering rigidly to routine can prevent the nursing team from managing care in a way which takes account of the individual needs of patients (Wells 1980, Pembrey 1980).

RECENT CHANGE

Writing in 1965 about ward sisters, Jenkinson suggested that as the Health Service settled down, sisters would be able to devote more attention to promotion of health, to education of staff and to research in addition to their primary responsibilities of caring for patients.

The Health Service has not settled down. Since 1965, major changes in the work roles and relationships of health professionals in hospital and community have directly and indirectly affected sisters.

For example, the implementation of the Salmon Committee's recommendations (MOH/SHHD 1966) on senior nursing staff structure directly influenced sisters, and of equal importance but perhaps less immediate impact has been debate about the Committee on Nursing's recommendations (DHSS 1972) for change in the education and training of nurses. There have also been two major reorganisations of the National Health Service, and the setting up of the United Kingdom Central Council for Nursing, Midwifery and Health Visiting has guaranteed that upheaval will continue as the Council and the four National Boards get down to reviewing and setting standards for education, training and professional conduct.

Industrial relations

Nurses are often criticised by their professional organisations for lack of sensitivity to major political and professional issues, and for lack of knowledge of important change; but there are undoubtedly many ways now in which government action has become real to sisters. For example, employment legislation reaches the ward. Many staff, including nurses, are members of trade unions. Staff appraisal and complaints about unsatisfactory performance or work conditions can no longer be dealt with according to personal whim by Matron. Delay in repair or maintenance of ward fabric remind a sister that the services of the hospital plumber, electrician or joiner, however willingly given, are subject to union rulings. On occasion, industrial action has been followed by improvements in conditions for patients and staff; but in the short term, disputes have disrupted ward management and directly hindered the provision of patient care.

Media interest

A further change has been the considerable increase in attention given by the media to professional practice and conduct. Achievement and error are now newsworthy.

In the 1920s the reason for a sister's dismissal did not even appear in the report of the Nursing Committee of her own hospital (Royal Infirmary of Edinburgh 1915–24). The fact of it alone was noted with brief comment which implied a breakdown in working relationships between the physician in charge and the sister, and a deterioration in the sister's mental state. The reader of the report is left to speculate about cause and effect.

By the 1970s, the dismissal and trial of a sister charged with murder and assault and her removal from the Register of the General Nursing Council for Scotland were matters for national debate and widely reported on radio, television and in newspapers (The Scotsman 1975). The Committee of Inquiry (Greater Glasgow Health Board 1975) for the incident scrutinised the nursing staff's problems, their range of responsibilities and the support available to them. The final report of the Committee of Inquiry suggested that many organisational changes, both in the hospital itself and in the National Health Service as a whole, had produced stress, understaffing and a lowering of morale. Other effects of the changes included remote management, poor communications and a failure to review conditions for patients and staff.

This particular case was complex, and debate about professional standards became mixed with legal wrangling. It did show, however, that sisters are directly affected by change and may require help to adapt to it. In order to adapt, they need to understand the nature of change and the effect it has on their work. It would seem that without adequate support, help and understanding, the physical and emotional cost of coping with change can be very high.

Sister and the team

As a result of changes in nursing and in society, sisters have become a mobile workforce and the increased turnover of trained staff has created considerable upheaval in hospitals (Redfern 1981).

Fifty years ago, there were few employment options available to trained nurses and promotion was slow. Today there are several careers in nursing and many specialised areas of work from which to choose.

Employment and career patterns have become influenced by factors such as marriage, child rearing and caring for other dependants (Hockey 1976). As a result, the amount of time which women in their early twenties and thirties spend in nursing has decreased and the needs of the nursing service have had to compete with choice of lifestyle and social commitments.

Reflecting changes in social climate, many sisters now have a dual role and few would consider hospital to be their home. The days when a sister worked, ate, relaxed and slept in hospital, and when students polished her grate, desk and brasses are now over.

Social and professional changes have also influenced others in the nursing team and a sister now faces a changing population, not just of learners, but of all grades of staff. There are many more part-time and unqualified members of staff; there have been cuts in the number of hours worked per week and the number of patients to be cared for has increased. As a result, pressures on sisters have risen and good communication within the team and continuity of care for patients have become more difficult to achieve.

Pattern of activity

In recent decades, many more people from inside and outside hospitals have become involved in patient care. Dieticians, physiotherapists and occupational therapists contribute to care; community health workers liaise between home and hospital and open visiting schemes give the public freer access to wards.

As a result, a sister now has to act as an expert co-ordinator and decision-maker at the centre of an increasingly complicated network of communications. She also has to try to protect patients from the potentially exhausting demands of frequent contact with many services, departments and exposure to unfamiliar faces.

These changes have altered the pattern and pace of sisters' activities and increased pressure on their time and on their reserves of energy. It has been found that most of a sister's activities on an average day last for less than a minute and that interruptions are a considerable problem (Davies 1972, Lelean 1973, Pembrey 1980). In an analysis of the movement of people in and out of a medical ward in a London teaching hospital over seven hours, it was noted that almost all of the 129 people who came into the ward consulted the ward sister (DHSS 1972, para 480).

McGhee (1961) neatly described the work of the sister as having been 'atomised'; and she suggested that fragmentation of work could be one cause of a sister's failure to establish good communications and good relationships.

Ward atmosphere and learning climate

McGhee (1961) also outlined the importance of the sister in determining 'ward atmosphere', which she defined as the state of relationships between staff and patients. Patients claimed a direct relationship between rate of recovery and good atmosphere.

To add to the link between sisters and 'atmosphere', there is now evidence of a relationship between sisters and the well-being of learners in a ward.

The sister is the key person who creates and controls the learning environment (Fretwell 1980) and it has been shown that 'ward learning climate' exists as a measurable reality for students (Orton 1981). From the learners' point of view, the most important elements in an ideal learning climate seem to be good teamwork and communications; the ideal sister is a skilled team leader who is seen to be caring and competent, democratic and approachable; she shows consideration towards her subordinates, is sensitive to trainees' needs, tries to motivate and involve them and give feedback on progress; she also makes a conscious effort to teach and in particular makes optimum use of ward report for teaching.

There are many difficulties inherent in the sister's teaching role. For example, sisters usually receive no preparation for this part of their work and the amount of time available for teaching can be very small. In Lelean's (1973) study of communication between sisters and nurses in six medical wards, the sisters spent very little time teaching and this was considered unsurprising in view of the fragmented, interrupted pattern of their work. The sisters in Lelean's study did communicate with nurses twice as frequently as those in

Revan's (1964) study, possibly because of the development of less authoritarian attitudes. However, Lelean found that only 3 per cent of the sister's informal communication was with first-year students. On most mornings there was no communication at all between the junior nurses and sister and when it did occur it tended to be one way only, from sister to learner.

Nurse management structure

Some praise and a great deal of criticism has been given to the revised senior nurse management structure which developed in hospitals after the extremely rapid implementation of the Salmon Committee's recommendations (Wall & Hespe 1972). For example, doctors warned of the possibility of problems such as devaluation of bedside nursing, overemphasis on promotion to administration, increasing numbers of young inexperienced sisters and erosion of ward sisters' duties (Anderson 1973, Nursing Times 1974). Since the 1960s, the working life of a sister has certainly shortened to around three years in that grade; but in 1974 doctors were reminded in a leading article in the British Medical Journal that the Salmon structure should not be made scapegoat for a whole range of social and professional factors which have created change (British Medical Journal 1974). Changes in women's role in society, in attitudes to work and working conditions and wider career choice have all contributed towards the disappearance of the faithful sister who spent most of her waking hours on the ward.

The Salmon structure has not devalued bedside nursing or taken increasing numbers of nurses from clinical areas into management; the numbers of nurses in administration has decreased in the last two decades (Gray & Smail 1981). It has been suggested, however, that Salmon has 'diverted attention and resources from the primary clinical role of the nurse' (McFarlane 1980, p. 18). The hierarchical management structure may be militating against the development of individual responsibility and initiative in providing direct patient care at ward level.

Sisters have criticised the present management structure for creating loss of self esteem and loss of autonomy, as being impersonal and complicated, and responsible for poor communications and delays in decision-making (Redfern 1981). Much of this dissatisfaction seems to be related to three interrelated factors: to the nature of the sister's relationship with her immediate superior, the nursing officer; to tensions between clinical and managerial components of nursing; and to difficulties dealing with the multiple authority relationship of sister with consultants and nursing officer.

It was envisaged originally that the nursing officer would deal with managerial matters such as staff deployment in the interests of efficient ward and unit management; she would act as a clinical consultant, advising ward staff on nursing practice, helping with patient care problems and developing new ideas; she would participate in the training of nursing staff including learners; and she would have a personnel function, providing support and dealing with staff appraisal and development. Sisters have levelled criticism at each part of the nursing officer's job, in particular at her failure to provide the right kind of support, at failure to act as clinical adviser on nursing problems and at failure to participate in teaching learners (Jones et al 1981). Heyman & Shaw (1980) found that included in reasons for 'annoyance with a nursing officer' were 'unwarranted interference, destructive criticism and lack of specialised knowledge' (p. 613).

The Royal Commission on the National Health Service (1979) pointed out that there are several reasons for the poor development of clinical and teaching aspects of the nursing officer's job. Expertise and special knowledge are quickly outdated without opportunities to practise and nursing officers have limited access to patients. The demands of management have left little time for clinical involvement and nursing officer training has emphasised management functions to the exclusion of preparation for an advanced clinical role. The nursing officer may be effectively excluded from teaching by the presence of a clinical teacher, and from clinical decision-making by the sister–consultant relationship.

Despite the tensions between sisters and nursing officers and the obvious difficulties of the nursing officer's job, some sisters have welcomed the improved long-term career opportunities in nurse management post-Salmon and better short-term opportunities to widen management experience. For other sisters, however, promotion to the nursing officer grade remains an unattractive prospect, the move 'into management' being perceived as a move 'out of nursing'.

Non-nursing duties

The Salmon Report (1966) and the Farrer Report (1968) recommended that nurses should be relieved of non-nursing duties, and schemes were introduced to free sisters from work which was considered inappropriate to the professional nurse. As a result, new relationship patterns have been developed between a sister and technical and ancillary staff.

In some hospitals, ward clerks were appointed supposedly to relieve sisters of paperwork and telephone calls. But the assumption that the introduction of clerical help eases the pressure on a sister has to be questioned. A ward clerk can be an invaluable figure in a ward team but she becomes one more person with whom the sister must regularly communicate. Pembrey (1980) found a higher number of perceived and observed interruptions for sisters in hospitals which had full-time ward clerks.

The ward clerk's usefulness will depend on many factors, such as whether there are claims on her services by other non-nursing members of staff, and whether she has knowledge and ability to use her discretion regarding the giving, seeking or withholding of information until the time is appropriate. It may also depend upon whether she uses her 'power' to facilitate communications or to block them. Ultimately the clerk's usefulness rests on the ability of the ward sister to integrate her into the scheme of ward management.

Another area of change has been the removal from nurses of control over 'hotel' services, such as catering, domestic cleaning, linen and laundry (Tolliday 1972). Sisters now face the problem of having to maintain interest in the level of efficiency of services over which they have no direct managerial control (Pembrey 1980).

Supervisors, nursing officers, clerks, receptionists and housekeepers have all become involved in helping to get service problems resolved; however, the loss of direct control has created the unsatisfactory situation where sister retains coordinating, monitoring and executive power at ward level for services, but can be divorced from involvement in planning and setting objectives for their change and improvement. To become involved, effective middle management support is needed; but if relationships and communications between sister and nursing officer are poor or ill-defined, then support may not be available, or may not be seen to be available. A sister may not be aware that objective setting is necessary; she may not realise that alternatives to the existing situation would be possible or preferable; she may not use existing opportunities to contribute to policy decisions, for example, at sisters' or unit meetings. In these situations, objectives may never be set, and static management with crisis intervention can become the rule.

Management training

Since 1966, when the Salmon Report recognised the need to prepare for a changing role, training for the sister's job has been provided mainly in the form of off-the-job courses. By trying to relate management principles to hospital organisation, courses have attempted to encourage sisters to think more objectively about their wards, to re-examine accepted situations and to increase awareness of opportunities to improve ward management. They have also tried to develop problem-solving ability, to increase self-confidence and understanding of relationships and behaviour, and to alter traditional ways of thinking.

There has been doubt, however, about the effectiveness of management training. Studies evaluating courses have highlighted many of the personal, professional and organisational problems experienced by sisters, and revealed some of the ways in which their problems have influenced and limited the effectiveness of the courses (Toman 1977). Davies (1972) found that, because of lack of pre-course preparation and post-course evaluation in hospital, sisters had no clear expectations of the management course or of the objectives they should achieve. The course occurred in a vacuum; it was enjoyed as 'time out' and as a pleasant break from routine but it was not regarded as particularly relevant. Sisters had difficulty in conceptualising, and in developing ideas and using information when back at work. Despite wishing to make changes, they often lacked incentive after the course was over, or lacked the social skills needed to implement change and were restricted by the organisational pattern within which they worked.

Many sisters were not accustomed to using their own initiative and did not understand their role as potential change agents. Often they failed to realise the complexity of situations; they looked for absolute, specific answers to problems and disliked experimenting with new ideas. Even when the complexity was realised and an attempt made to analyse it, well-tried routines remained preferable as the safe response; change which upset routine was threatening and avoided.

It is also interesting that Davies (1972) labelled many of the sisters' comments as 'ritual' in nature; for example, she suggested that when talking about 'the importance of good communications', sisters were simply using a phrase common in the hospital culture. Despite their use of such remarks, many sisters lacked self-awareness and insight into their own attitudes and behaviour.

In her conclusion Davies suggests that management courses do have a part to play in helping a sister to understand her working environment, and to develop a more positive approach to problems which affect her, but which are outside her immediate control. Her study focuses on the interplay of the individual and the organisation; but it does not highlight the importance of management principles and techniques in relation to the management of nursing as distinct from the management of the complex ward environment. The two aspects of management are interdependent (Williams & Message 1969), but Davies (1972) does not emphasise the central function of the sister as manager of a nursing team whose objective is the assessment, planning, implementation and evaluation of care for individual patients.

In contrast, Pembrey's study (1980) focused on the role of the sister in the management of nursing itself. Most sisters in a sample of 50 were found to spend little time on 'management of nursing activities'. It seemed that the daily nursing of patients was not actively managed but tended to be governed by ward and hospital routine.

Seven out of the 50, however, were identified as 'manager' sisters. These sisters were able to organise nursing on an individual patient basis through the completion of a four step 'nursing management cycle'; they defined work by doing a nursing round of patients; they prescribed work verbally and in writing; they delegated authority to work to nursing teams responsible for groups of patients; and they exacted accountability for work by receiving reports from team leaders on each patient. These sisters were found to be the most highly qualified academically and professionally of the sample; they also considered that their management training had been inappropriate for their job as sister. They felt that they had learned how to manage the nursing from watching and working with other sisters; in other words, from experienced role models rather than from formal management courses.

As a result of a rethink about the potential value of role models and because of increasing concern about the inadequacy of management courses, experimental training wards for sisters have now been set up and are currently being evaluated (King's Fund Project Report 1981). These ward-based schemes aim to use experienced sisters as role models to teach future sisters.

Off-the-job courses can help with professional development and can act as a stimulus towards change, provided that organisational support is available and that course objectives are seen to be relevant to the reality of the sister's own ward and hospital. It has been found that when the active involvement of the sister's immediate superior, the nursing officer, is obtained for pre- and post-course training discussion, the effectiveness of management training increases and improved job performance occurs (White & Frawley 1975).

Management audit

Attempts have been made to monitor nursing performance by using systems of audit. Management audit focuses on administrative aspects of a nurse's responsibilities with the objective of improving the quality of management and nursing care (Huczynski 1977, Elliott & Fisher 1979).

In his evaluation of the management audit used in Doncaster, in which most participants were at sister level, Huczynski (1977) identified a number of benefits and drawbacks in the system. After completing an audit form, each nurse discussed in detail with her immediate superior her responses to questions and statements about all aspects of nursing management. Included in the audit were attempts to identify problem areas and to set goals and long-term objectives with superiors. It was found that most nurses regarded the identification of problem areas as the primary objective of the audit; sisters, however, did not value highly opportunities to set long-term objectives and monitor progress, and many ended their interview with their nursing officer without agreeing work targets or key tasks for the future. Some of the sisters believed that the problems identified would be solved by the nursing officer.

It was concluded that establishing the audit on the basis of 'getting the problems solved' was not a sound idea; 'the majority of benefits identified by participants had little to do with problem-solution, but focused on personal growth, increased motivation and improved interpersonal relationships. It was in these fields that it was strongest' (Huczynski 1977, p. 529). It would seem that goal setting and learning about the pitfalls of problem solving are important topics for sisters and their nursing officers to consider.

Isolation

In such a complex work environment, surrounded by so many people, it may seem a contradiction to suggest that sisters are isolated. It was mentioned earlier that authoritarianism can isolate but nowadays there are other forms of isolation which sisters experience as a result of changes in patterns of ward work and in colleague relationships. For example, geographical isolation within a ward or hospital environment has changed. The sister who used to 'live in' was isolated to some extent from the community; she could identify readily with the 'us' of ward staff and patients and with the wider hospital environment which was home, but perhaps less readily with the 'them' of the community which included patients' relatives and friends. Now, reflecting the splitting of private and professional identities, a sister is likely to identify with ward and community but perhaps less readily with the wider hospital environment. As the organisational structure of hospitals has become more complicated, the overall picture of how they function has blurred and the focus of work has narrowed to the ward. Hospital notice boards point to unknown departments whose function is obscure. Lack of involvement in the wider hospital environment or even lack of curiosity about it can limit the sister's ability to use fully the services which it provides.

Turning the focus of activities in upon a ward can also hinder the development of contact with what Davies (1972) calls the 'colleague reference group', that is, other sisters. Davies suggests that interrupted career patterns and job mobility have resulted in colleague relationships being regarded as less important. Contact with sister colleagues nowadays may be infrequent and limited to the dining room, the telephone or the occasional sisters' or unit meeting.

Problems of conflicting loyalties can also isolate a sister. For example, in a situation of acute staff shortage, a consultant might plead the case to nursing administration for more nursing staff. Even if the consultant's request is based on genuinely perceived need, the nursing hierarchy might resent the doctor's request, interpreting it as interference in a nursing matter or as manipulative behaviour on the part of the ward sister using medical support to increase pressure for a larger share of limited resources. If the sister relies too heavily on the consultant's help, she might find herself avoiding action which could displease him or lead him to withdraw his support. The displeasure of nursing superiors can be obvious or subtle. Where there is defensiveness, mistrust or unsatisfactory communications, there will be extra tension; in a tangle of relationships with conflicting loyalties, the sister may well find herself isolated in the midst of sectional interests.

Fear of being isolated can lead to pressure to conform. If a sister upsets the status quo, the label 'troublemaker' might be applied by her own nursing team or by her nursing superiors; if her ideas are rejected, she might conform rather than find herself ignored, criticised, victimised or isolated. Pembrey (1980) found that sisters who tried to innovate and introduce new ideas felt isolated and unsupported. Loneliness, isolation and lack of personal support for sisters were also noted by Cortazzi & Roote (1975) in their analysis of ward team problems; they suggest that the question 'Who supports the nurse?' is urgently in need of examination.

2

Sister and her role

Theories from many disciplines have been used widely in the study of nurses and other health workers (Chapman 1976, McFarlane 1977). In this chapter, the sister's work and some of its problems are looked at from the point of view of role theory.

Banton (1965) has suggested that analysing interactions and social relationships in terms of roles 'brings some sort of order into the contemplation of the bewildering complexity of human activities' (p. 38). In the early stages of this study, certain concepts from role theory helped to inject some 'order' into the author's thinking about the complexities of her own and colleagues' experiences as sisters. The limitations of using existing theory, however, had to be recognised; one danger being that reality can be oversimplified by adopting a theory in such a way that complex behaviour and observations are made to fit existing concepts. This study was not designed, therefore, solely within the framework of role theory.

ROLE

The position which a sister holds in the organisational structure of a ward and a hospital is associated with a particular pattern of expected behaviour. The sister's role is related to other people's ideas about what she should do, that is, norms; it is related to other people's ideas about what they expect her to do, that is, expectations; and it is related to her own ideas about what she should do, that is, self-expectations. Role is more than a description of a sister's behaviour. It is the cluster of functions, obligations and duties expected of her as she plays her part in the hospital organisation.

Merton (1957a) has suggested that control is exerted on behaviour in three main ways: first, through clearly defined rules or laws which specify what one must do; second, through less clearly defined expectations held by self and by others regarding what one ought to do; and third, through habit, custom and routine. These three elements of control are evident in the work of the sister. For example, a sister must see that rules governing the safe custody of drugs are adhered to; a consultant may expect a sister to be present at all his rounds; and a sister might routinely carry out a round of the patients after coming on duty.

ROLE-SET

Merton (1957b) recognised that one person may be confronted with an array of roles and expectations and he used the term 'role-set' to describe the network of relationships which surround a role.

Figure 1 illustrates a sister's role-set and shows the many people with whom she interacts. In a ward, the network of complementary roles and relationships is wide and the sets of expectations complex and changing. Individuals and groups within the role-set may have different interests and values; there may be differences between them in amount of contact and degree of involvement with sister and in opportunities to observe and understand each other's work; there may also be differences between them in the distribution of power and authority (Davies 1972).

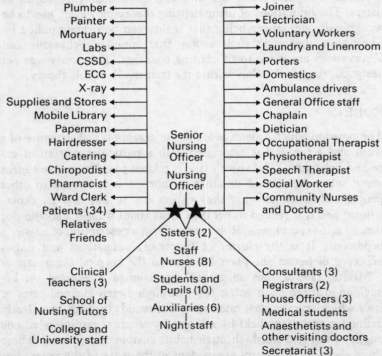

Figure 1 A ward sister's role-set (the author's)

Expectations may be clear and reinforce each other but they can also be unclear and may provide a basis for confusion, conflict and dissatisfaction. In an American study of social and psychological factors which affect nursing performance, Benne & Bennis (1959) outlined some aspects of confusion in the role of the nurse and suggested four main sets of expectations which determine the nurse role:

Institutional expectations from those in the administrative hierarchy

Expectations from all colleagues in the ward team, such as nurses, doctors and paramedical staff

Expectations from reference groups outside the work situation, such as family, church, professional associations, and the nurse's own training school or college

The nurse's self-expectations of what she should be and do.

Patients are a notable omission from this classification but they are included in Chapman's (1976) simple diagram which shows patients, relatives, public, colleagues, paramedical staff and doctors as the principal groups with whom the nurse interacts. After describing some of the many different kinds of behaviour which these groups would expect of a nurse, Chapman concludes: 'No wonder that the nurse feels that she has to be all things to all men and that she occasionally gets her responses to expected behaviour mixed' (p. 113).

CONFLICT

Several forms of conflict can be experienced by sisters.

Inter-role conflict

When a person simultaneously occupies two or more roles — for example, wife and ward sister — the demands of the roles may be incompatible and conflict can occur. As social life has become increasingly complex, the incidence of conflict between roles has risen. A sister might experience this type of conflict when aspects of her work role, such as having to work late or having to take paperwork home, become incompatible with the demands of family and social commitments.

Intra-role conflict

Each group with whom a sister works is likely to develop expectations more attuned to its own organisational values than to those of the sister. Intra-role conflict occurs when people who work with a sister have different expectations about how she should behave. For example, a sister may not agree with a consultant's expectations that she should be present at all his ward rounds.

This form of conflict is one outcome of having to maintain working relationships with a wide variety of complementary roles. Studies in educational, industrial and health care settings suggest that the greater the diversity of a role-set, the greater the chance of conflict within a role (Hansen & Upshaw 1962, Kahn & Wolfe 1964, Snoek 1966).

Self-role conflict

Behaviour is influenced not only by the expectations of others, but also by self-expectations.

Self-role conflict occurs when there is discrepancy between what the nurse expects of herself and her actual behaviour, that is, between what she would like to be and the reality of what she is and does.

Lack of fit between self-image and work has been called 'role deprivation' (Benne & Bennis 1959). The image of 'real nursing' as bedside care is one commonly held by the general public. From this, the student nurse begins to develop her expectations of the nurse role. If training and practical experience consistently reinforce the view that it is direct nursing care which is 'real nursing', then problems of conflict can occur when registered nurses have to deal with many other duties perceived as 'not real nursing'. There is evidence that some sisters regard giving direct nursing care as the most important part of their job. A commonly held view among sisters in Redfern's (1981) study was that a sister would want to do what she felt she had been trained to do: 'to nurse patients herself, rather than to act as an organiser, co-ordinator and superviser in delivering individualised care to the patient' (p. 83). The sister who bemoans the fact that it is weeks since she rolled up her sleeves 'to do a bed-bath' may be expressing some of her conflict between her idealistic and realistic images of nursing. If nurses select work because they like to respond to dependency, then they may experience conflict and tension when they find that nursing has to be redefined to fit contexts other than that of bedside nursing of dependent patients.

Role strain

Some writers consider role conflict to be simply one of several elements which together produce strain and pressure in a role (Kahn et al 1964).

Role strain can be experienced as:

1. *Conflict*, from incompatible expectations
2. *Overload*, when demands from many groups pile up beyond the worker's capacity, creating the problem of having to deal with conflicts between priorities. Sorting out conflicts between priorities is made more difficult if groups do not share the same view of the importance of tasks or are unaware of each other's expectations
3. *Ambiguity*, when there is lack of clear information about what is expected of a worker and uncertainty about the outcome of work and job performance. Information may not be available, it might not be communicated or it could be deliberately restricted.

Redfern (1981) used a number of role stress measures in her study of the job attitudes and occupational stability of sisters. Nearly three-quarters of her sample of 134 sisters experienced moderate or high levels of role conflict and job-related tension. Conflict arose from having to work with many groups which operated differently and from receiving incompatible requests. Some sisters experienced ambiguity because they were uncertain about their responsibilities, about the limits of their authority and about how their work was evaluated by the nursing officers. Others felt that they had very little control over decisions made by management.

Kahn & Wolfe (1964) identified factors which affect and modify role pressure, such as personality, position in the organisational hierarchy, autonomy and interpersonal relationships. They found that pressures from trusted associates seemed to arouse less tension. Trust and respect encouraged shared problem-solving, and this was more likely to occur when the need for change in a situation or an individual was seen to be acceptable to all concerned. When pressure was strong, the workers experienced more tension and futility, less job satisfaction and less confidence in the organisation; pressure was 'expensive to an organisation in terms of the morale of the role performer' (p. 119).

Adapting to conflict

There are many ways of responding to role demands and of adapting to problems of conflict, overload, or ambiguity. For example, a sister might try to inject change into her work situation and alter role relationships persuading others to change or modify their demands; she might herself try to change so that her image of her role and her personality fit the demands of the organisation more closely; she might try to shut off or block communication with others, aggravating the situation by increasing the pressure on those trying to communicate with her; she could try to avoid anxiety and stress by using defence mechanisms to distort the reality of situations (Menzies 1960); she might try to retain power and authority rather than delegate; she could take it out on family and friends outwith the work situation; she might stay and appear to comply but in fact withdraw psychologically, working apathetically and meeting only minimal work requirements; or she might leave her post.

The author recalls colleagues' conflicts with medical staff over requests for nurses to be responsible for the cardiac monitoring of patients in an open medical ward. It was felt that effective monitoring required continuous, or very frequent, observation of machine and patient to note changes in general condition and in heart rate and rhythm. In a general ward, as distinct from a coronary care unit, there was seldom a suitably trained nurse available to use the machine and to interpret changes on the oscilloscope. Sisters dealt with this in different ways. Some refused to be responsible, pointing out that under such staffing circumstances monitoring would be false security for patient and doctor, and might be an anxiety provoker for patient and nurses. Those who accepted the responsibility under protest dealt with the dilemma in various ways: some ignored or denied the problem; some used the presence of the monitor as an excuse for demanding more staff as though to 'nurse the machine'; some buried their feelings, reluctantly obeyed the orders and 'inwardly burned'. Benne & Bennis (1959) suggest that concealing conflict behind 'a bland mask of compliance' can 'levy a toll upon the nurse's personal adjustment, and the basic effectiveness and efficiency of the organisation suffer' (p. 198).

Coping responses can be useful and are sometimes essential to meet the needs and pressures of the moment, but on balance they are more likely to be inefficient and costly to an individual and the organisation (Wolfe & Snoek 1962).

Boulding (1964) points out that it may be unrealistic to talk about the resolution of conflict. The word resolution has an air of finality about it and it might be more appropriate to think in terms of conflict management rather than conflict resolution, the objective of conflict management being to make it creative and useful rather than destructive.

If used constructively, conflict can have positive outcomes and clash of values and interests between what is and what ought to be can exert pressure towards innovation and creativity (Coser 1967). Innovation implies the introduction of something new and the making of changes; creativity, although similar, suggests the bringing into being of something essentially new rather than the application of existing ways to new situations. But before conflict can be creatively harnessed in the interests of change, it must be recognised and understood; and it must be asked whether sisters see themselves as change agents, as being able to respond positively to conflict in wards and hospitals where the pressure may well be towards maintaining predictability and reducing anxiety, through habit, routine and ritual.

3

Sample, design and methods

The purpose of the study was to identify problems experienced by ward sisters and to examine the sisters' perceptions of their difficulties at work. Early in the study several problem areas were found from conversations with sisters, from review of the literature, and during exploratory, in-depth interviews with eight sisters in general medical and surgical wards. From these interviews several factors emerged which influenced the study design.

It was found that each sister could identify readily her work difficulties and each seemed keen to talk about them, often at length. When asked to talk about problems or pressures experienced on the day of interview or the previous day, the sisters could richly illustrate their difficulties. There was broad agreement about the types of problems experienced, but the initial list was not exhaustive as each sister identified new worries. It also quickly became apparent that similar problems were perceived differently and that sisters had varying degrees of insight into the nature of their problems.

For all these reasons, it was decided to continue the exploratory approach by carrying out in-depth case studies of a small group of sisters, further comparing and categorising problem areas, and exploring the various perceptions of problems.

SAMPLE

The study was carried out in Scotland in two district general hospitals of similar size (500 to 600 beds), one a city hospital, the other rural. Both hospitals provided facilities for the training of student and pupil nurses and medical students.

Nine sisters from seven wards participated, four sisters in the pilot study hospital and five in the main study hospital. Tables 3.1 and 3.2 identify the sisters and the characteristics of their medical and surgical wards.

22

Table 3.1   Pilot study: Sisters, type of post and ward characteristics

Sister	Type of post	Type of ward	No. of beds	Ward design
Green	Single sister	Surgical	20	Nightingale
Gold	Single sister	Medical/surgical	25	Divided
Blue	Single sister	Medical	34	Divided
Red	Shared — two sisters	Medical	58	Divided

Table 3.2   Main study: Sisters, type of post and ward characteristics

Sister	Type of post	Type of ward	No. of beds	Ward design
Grey	Shared — two sisters	Medical	25	Nightingale
Brown White }	Shared — two sisters	Medical	25	Nightingale
Black Pink }	Shared — two sisters	Surgical	26	Nightingale

Background information

Each sister completed a questionnaire giving information about age, marital status, general educational attainment, professional qualifications and experience and future career plans (Tables 3.3 and 3.4).

In the pilot study hospital the four sisters were unmarried and planned to continue in nursing, expressing interest in moving to health visiting or clinical teaching. In terms of numbers and grades of certificates held, these sisters had higher levels of academic attainment than the main study sisters. There was a tendency for all the pilot study sisters to be more actively involved in continuing education than the main study sisters; one sister held the Diploma in Nursing and two were studying for Part B of the Diploma.

In the main study hospital all sisters were married. One planned to seek promotion to nurse management, four expected to remain in their present posts and one considered leaving nursing mainly because of dissatisfaction with pay and conditions of service.

Each sister was asked to note the number of medical staff using the ward and the number and grade of nursing staff available to her. The sisters also wrote down an outline of their day's work indicating those aspects which they considered priorities.

Using a semi-structured interview, information was obtained about medical specialties and bed use; each sister was also asked for her views about ward design, services and maintenance, about frequency of contact with nursing officer and clinical teacher, about

Table 3.3 Pilot study sisters: Age, marital status, educational attainment and professional experience

Sister	Age years	Marital status	Educational attainment*			No. of years in nursing	No. of years as sister	No. of professional qualifications
			2–5 'O'	6+ 'O'	H or 'A'			
Green	26–30	Single		✓		10	2	2
Gold	31–35	Single		✓	✓	14	4	4
Blue	31–35	Single		✓	✓	11	3	4
Red	31–35	Single	✓			13	7	4

*'O' = O Levels   H = Scottish Highers   'A' = A Levels

Table 3.4 Main study sisters: Age, marital status, educational attainment and professional experience

Sister	Age years	Marital status	Educational attainment*			No. of years in nursing	No. of years as sister	No. of professional qualifications
			2–5 'O'	6+ 'O'	H or 'A'			
Grey	31–35	Married			✓	12	5	2
Brown	41–45	Married		✓		8	3	1
White	26–30	Married		✓		8	3	2
Black	31–35	Married	✓			12	5	3
Pink	21–25	Married			✓	5	1	1

*'O' = O Levels   H = Scottish Highers   'A' = A Levels

her attendance at unit or other meetings and about any other professional commitments undertaken within or outside her hospital.

STUDY DESIGN

The study was conducted in two parts, first 'on-the-job' and second 'off-the-job'.

On-the-job

Three methods were used: observation, the semantic differential and interview.

Each sister was observed using direct, non-participant continuous observation for two morning sessions each 4½ hours, for two afternoon sessions each 4 hours and for two evening sessions each 5½ hours, a total of 28 hours. The six periods covered different days of the week and included at least one ward round morning; because the sisters suggested that the pace of work differed on Saturdays and Sundays, two periods out of six were observed at weekends.

At the end of each shift, an attempt was made to get a picture of how the sister felt or perceived herself during the observed period by using the semantic differential, an objective measure of self-perception. This involved completing four cards. Each card contained a different 'stimulus' concept and the same ten adjective pairs or rating scales (Fig. 2). The four concepts rated on these scales were:

Myself today as ward sister
Myself today with the patients
Myself today with the nurses
Myself today with the doctors.

The cards were completed very quickly, within 2 to 4 minutes. Each sister was then interviewed and asked the following questions about the period during which she had been observed. The interviews lasted from 15 to 30 minutes.

1. How would you describe the morning/afternoon/evening?
   Would you say it was good, bad or average; why would you describe it that way?
   Would you say it was busy, quiet or average; why would you describe it that way?
2. You spent time with many people today. How do you feel about the time you spent with the patients, with the nurses, with the doctors, with others?

MYSELF TODAY AS WARD SISTER

Sister ....
Day ....

Disapproving	- - - : - - - : - - - : - - - : - - - : - - - : - - -	Approving
Organised	- - - : - - - : - - - : - - - : - - - : - - - : - - -	Disorganised
Passive	- - - : - - - : - - - : - - - : - - - : - - - : - - -	Active
Uninfluential	- - - : - - - : - - - : - - - : - - - : - - - : - - -	Influential
Calm	- - - : - - - : - - - : - - - : - - - : - - - : - - -	Irritable
Attentive	- - - : - - - : - - - : - - - : - - - : - - - : - - -	Inattentive
Harmful	- - - : - - - : - - - : - - - : - - - : - - - : - - -	Beneficial
Sociable	- - - : - - - : - - - : - - - : - - - : - - - : - - -	Unsociable
Strong	- - - : - - - : - - - : - - - : - - - : - - - : - - -	Weak
Satisfied	- - - : - - - : - - - : - - - : - - - : - - - : - - -	Dissatisfied

Figure 2 Semantic differential

3. Did you have any problems today as ward sister? If yes, what were they?
4. Did you feel under pressure at any time today? If yes, what was happening at the time?
5. In what way could the day's work have been improved for you?

It can be seen that question 2 was related directly to the semantic differential concepts.

At the end of the 'on-the-job' study each sister completed four additional semantic differential cards, using again the same adjective pairs; the concepts rated were:

Sister as clinician
Sister as teacher
Sister as manager
The ideal sister.

Off-the-job

Two to three weeks later, the second part of the study was carried out. Each sister was interviewed 'off-the-job', when out of the ward and free from the pressure of immediate work constraints. On this occasion, work problems were examined using 25 cards each containing one problem statement. Each sister first gave every statement a 'worry' rating on a five-point scale, then ranked the 25 problems in order from 1 to 25 in terms of greatest (1) to least (25) worry. Finally the sister was invited to talk about her experiences and views about each problem, giving reasons for her rating and rank ordering and the interviews were tape recorded. Two interviews lasted approximately 30 minutes, four lasted approximately 1 hour, two lasted 1½ hours, but Sister Grey characteristically completed hers in the same manner as all other observed work, at high speed and in 15 minutes.

In the pilot study, all methods were tested with Sisters Gold and Green. Sisters Blue and Red, who worked in the larger wards, were not observed or interviewed 'on-the-job'; they participated only in the 'off-the-job' interviews, testing the use of the 25 problem statements. Since the latter method remained unchanged in the main study and because their interviews (1½ hours) so richly illustrated the nature of the job and its dilemmas, the remarks of these two sisters have been included in the analysis of the 25 problems in Chapter 5.

METHODS

Observation

To provide information about the content and pattern of the sisters' activities against which interview and semantic differential data could be examined, observation was used to answer the following questions: What does Sister do? How much time does she spend on each activity? How much time does she spend with patients, nurses and doctors? Who initiates her activities? How often is she interrupted? How fragmented is her activity? And, where in the ward or hospital does she spend her time?

To record the pattern and fragmentation of activity, continuous observation rather than activity sampling was necessary; a non-participant observer role was adopted.

Activity code list

Following exploratory work, a code list of 36 ward sister activities was drawn up (Appendix 1). Existing lists, used in work study and work measurement, were felt to be inappropriate and unnecessarily detailed (Goddard 1953).

The code list was developed with help from a research assistant, a nurse tutor. The author and her assistant independently observed two sisters and recorded their activities by describing them in words in as much detail as time allowed. The described activities were categorised and coded and further observation was then carried out to check whether codes and categories were mutually exclusive and exhaustive. The five main categories were: activities with patients; activities with the nursing team; activities with doctors; activities with nurse managers and other hospital personnel; and general administration.

As a reliability check the activities of one sister were simultaneously but independently observed by the researcher and her assistant and the results of coding compared; a high measure of agreement was obtained.

The help of the tutor colleague, who observed the sisters using a different frame of reference, was valuable for checking bias, inferences and selective perception. For example, an interaction between a sister and a nurse was described by the tutor as teaching and by the author as a work order. On discussion it was decided that although a teaching/learning opportunity could have been said to exist, there was no observable evidence within that unit of behaviour that teaching and learning had occurred; also, there were other elements such as social conversation in the contact in addition to the giving of an order, therefore the contact was coded simply as 'Talking with nurses'.

During the pilot and main studies, all observation was conducted by only one observer, therefore inferences and interpretations were unchecked.

Unit of behaviour

Exploratory observation confirmed the author's hunch that detailed recording of all that a sister did would prove difficult. The sisters responded to sensory cues and changed the focus of their attention so rapidly that it was sometimes impossible to document quickly enough all the very brief segments of behaviour as they occurred; the sisters were also often observed doing more than one thing at a time. For example, a sister was observed to answer one phone, to ask the caller to wait while she answered the second phone; while talking to the second caller, she made an entry in the nursing Kardex and filed papers in her desk; she asked the second caller to wait while she talked briefly to a patient's relatives, inviting them to take a seat in her room; she then gave a passing nurse a work order, completed the second phone conversation and returned to the first phone call and all this occurred within one minute. During this, she had apparently also become aware of a patient calling from the ward area, since on completing the first phone call and before talking to the relatives, she excused herself, remarking, 'I must see Mr X . . . .'

It was not possible, therefore, to use as a unit of behaviour the smallest observable segment of verbal or non-verbal behaviour observed; rather, because of the complexity of detail, as many shifts of attention as possible from person to person or activity to activity were recorded within one minute. Where activities occurred together or in very quick succession, as many as possible were noted in sequence.

Using a digital watch, the starting time of each activity was recorded.

All the variables observed were coded: for example the activity itself; the initiator of the activity; the location of the activity; and the people with whom sister was involved. Patients, nurses and doctors were given individual codes.

A recording form was designed from which data could be punched directly and stored on disc for computer processing. In retrospect, complex computer processing was inappropriate and a simpler form of analysis could have been used. For those interested in further detail about the coding and the form used, more information is available in the thesis on which this book is based (Runciman 1980).

Interruptions

Exploratory observation highlighted the problem of defining and recording interruptions in sisters' activities. Sisters were often interrupted in the sense that other people or telephone calls made them stop what they were doing; often, however, the sisters interrupted themselves.

A single activity, such as writing up the nursing Kardex in the evening, could begin at 19.00 hours and end at 21.30 hours with sister making many brief stabs at its completion. From the sisters' remarks, it was clear that not all intervening activities were felt to be interruptions, and the same type of intervening activity could be perceived as an interruption on one occasion but not on another. Observation as a tool for recording interruptions was, therefore, limited, and the sisters' own comments were necessary to throw light on the ways in which interruptions were perceived and defined.

It was possible, however, to obtain some quantitative data about the interruption factor when the term interruption was defined as an intervening unit of behaviour which broke the continuity of another main activity whose start and finish could be identified. For example, a nursing report session, a drug round or a consultant's round had an identifiable beginning and end, and for these activities, interruptions were identified.

Non-participant observer role

The non-participant observer role was discussed with each sister before starting and a 30-minute trial period of observation carried out to allow the sister to see what was involved and to say how she felt about being watched; this also allowed the researcher to select unobtrusive observation points and to become familiar with ward layout.

The effect of the sisters' involvement in the study upon their behaviour — the Hawthorne effect — had to be considered (Treece & Treece 1977). Changes in the behaviour of nurses while being observed tend to be in a positive direction and any attempts to improve performance are therefore usually considered to be acceptable (Hall 1978, Watson 1979). All sisters remarked that observation had not bothered them and that generally they were too busy to notice the observer. On several occasions when wards were very quiet, the sisters did not feel that they had to keep busy, and the author was invited to sit with them, have tea or join in social conversation. The percentage of time spent talking with the researcher remained at an acceptably low level and ranged from 0.2 to 2.0 per cent. Meal breaks were taken with sisters at their invitation; no recordings were made at these times despite the fact that the sisters kept working during their breaks, seizing opportunities to talk to people in the dining room or in corridors.

Although being observed did not appear to worry or to influence the behaviour of the sisters unduly, there were times when acting as observer of ward activities was an uncomfortable experience. An example of such an occasion, when the author felt ill at ease, and when the non-participant observer role was difficult to sustain, is described in the next chapter.

Semantic differential

The semantic differential technique was developed by Osgood and his colleagues (1957) as a measure of the meaning of concepts. It was used in this study to examine the meaning of self concepts. Warr & Knapper (1968) suggested that there are three main factors which influence judgements of self — attributive, expectancy and affective factors. A sister might attribute to herself certain characteristics, such as adaptability; she might expect certain behaviour of herself, such as being organised; and she might respond emotionally to her own behaviour, for example with approval or disapproval. The semantic differential provides insight into self judgements of covert characteristics and is a measure of the three aspects of person perception.

A semantic differential consists of a number of seven point rating scales applied to a series of adjective pairs. Given a set of scales, subjects rate a concept on every scale in turn, the term concept referring to the 'stimulus' to which the subject checks his 'response'. Constructing a semantic differential requires selection of adjective pairs and concepts which are relevant to the subject being studied.

Scales — adjective pairs

Osgood and his colleagues found that adjective pairs fall into clusters. Using factor analysis, they identified three main factors or dimensions of meaning: first, an evaluative factor, as in adjective pairs good—bad, pleasant—unpleasant; second, a potency or strength factor, as in strong—weak; and third, an activity factor as in active—passive.

To cover these dimensions of meaning, ten adjective pairs were chosen, representing the three factors (Fig. 2). The order in which the scales were presented and the position of positive–negative adjectives were randomly assigned.

In selecting the scales, the influence of 'social desirability' was taken into account since responses distorted in the direction of social desirability are a possible source of biased error (Heise 1969). It had to be considered, for example, whether a sister would ever give negative ratings to certain adjectives such as bad, weak or disorganised, or indeed whether she would ever positively rate herself as good. It was found that there was a tendency to avoid negative scores on the beneficial–harmful scale; it could be that the choice of this adjective pair was unsatisfactory since harmful might have been considered an undesirable response.

Concepts

The eight concepts were selected by another group of sisters on the basis of their relevance to the job. It was felt that the concepts chosen would elicit a range of response from the study sisters and would be familiar and readily understood.

It could be argued that the function concepts of manager, teacher and clinician were not mutually exclusive, but their selection was felt to be justified because in writing about the sister's work the manager, teacher, clinician framework tends to be adopted and because sisters themselves use these terms to distinguish facets of their role; facets which, in exploratory interviews, were found to be viewed and valued differently.

Each concept with its set of scales was presented on a separate card and the order of presentation of the cards was randomised. The instructions for use were based on those of Osgood et al (1957).

Scoring

The semantic differential was analysed in several ways. Scale positions were assigned scores from 1 to 7; 1 identified the negative end point, 7 the positive end point, and 4 the neutral position. With 10 scales per concept, the maximum concept score was $7 \times 10 = 70$.

The concept scores and the individual scale scores were examined each day in relation to the sister's remarks when interviewed and it was found that the scores did validate the sisters' comments.

Using D scores, or distance scores, the relationship between certain concepts was also examined (Kerlinger 1965). The smaller the D score the more alike the concepts, the greater the D score the more unalike the concepts. Scores for the concepts of the manager, the teacher, the clinician, the ideal sister and the self as sister were compared.

The semantic differential did succeed in providing insights into the sisters' perceptions of self from day-to-day and in their work role in general. The concepts and scales seemed to have face validity, the sisters had no difficulty completing the cards and there were no rating omissions or errors. The technique also proved to have the major advantages of being quick to administer and easy to complete.

Problem statements — rating, ranking and interview

Personal experience, review of the literature and exploratory interviews provided a collection of problem statements from which the following themes emerged: lack of time; lack of staff; interruptions; student nurses; patients; doctors; stores, supplies and maintenance; ward management; and workload. There is some similarity between these themes and Pembrey's (1980) five categories of work problems: ward services and maintenance; interruptions; admission and discharge policy; medical staff; nursing resources.

Using the sisters' own words whenever possible, a list of 25 problem statements was drawn up. They are arranged here in the seven categories in which they are analysed in Chapter 5:

Sister and the patients
Having enough contact with patients
Finding time to talk with the patients in a leisurely way
Doing basic nursing care
Finding out whether the work is being done

Sister and the learners
Having enough contact with the student nurses
Teaching the student nurses

Sister as coordinator
Being interrupted so often
Being available to everyone while on duty
Meeting the demands of so many people
Not having enough time to myself while on duty
Feeling tired
Doing ward work in off-duty time
Having too much to do every day
Doing things that are not part of my job
Friction between staff

Sister and the nursing officer
Getting the nursing officer to understand the ward
Finding someone to turn to when I need help

Sister and the doctors
Disagreeing with a doctor's instructions for a patient
Getting the doctors to listen to my point of view

Learning the job
Considering myself as a manager
Understanding my job responsibilities
Getting the staff nurses to understand the ward sister's role

Keeping up to date
Keeping up to date with new trends
Feeling isolated from other ward sisters
Making changes in the ward

Numbers were randomly assigned to the statements and the list reordered to reduce the chance of category rather than statement response.

There were three steps in the rating and ranking procedure which was completed within 5 to 10 minutes. The cards were first rated in three categories, then rated in five categories representing greatest to least areas of 'worry'. Finally they were ranked from 1 to 25 representing greatest to least problem. There was no difficulty using the forced-choice method of ranking and there were no tied rank placements. The tape-recorded interviews based on the statements were transcribed and their content analysed in the context of all the other information obtained from each sister.

4

Problems found on the job

PILOT STUDY

Drawing together information from the interview after each shift, from the semantic differentials and from observation, this chapter presents an on-the-job profile of each sister. The profiles describe the problems which the sisters experienced, the situations which created pressures, possible improvements to the day and the ingredients which made the days good or bad, busy or quiet.

Sister Gold (Table 4.1)

Instructing doctors
The problems on both mornings concerned the doctors. Sister Gold had spent a considerable amount of time teaching a new doctor and a medical student about preparation and administration of certain drugs, matters which she felt should have been dealt with by senior medical staff. The medical cover was described as 'totally inadequate'. The concept Self with doctors had the lowest score for this day.

Information overload
On the 'bad, busy' morning, which had the lowest total semantic differential (SD) score, Sister Gold said there was 'an awful lot of work to get through' and she felt 'disorganised'. She had been off for two days and the staff nurse who had been on duty then was not available to tell her what had been happening in the ward. Much new information had to be 'straightened out' in her mind and the lack of continuity created a feeling of pressure.

Similar numbers of observed activities were recorded on the 'bad, busy' and the 'good, quiet' mornings. The activity pattern of the 'bad' morning was more fragmented with 48 per cent of activities lasting less than one minute compared with 37 per cent on the good morning. The latter was 'good' because sister felt 'organised from the start', 'everything went to plan', 'there were no crises',

35

Table 4.1 Sister Gold. Daily profiles — problems, pressure and improvements. Medical ward, 25 beds.

	Morning	Morning*	Afternoon*	Afternoon	Evening	Evening
Description of the day	Good Quiet	Bad Busy	Average Average	Good Quiet	Average Busy	Average Busy
Problems experienced	Yes	Yes	—	—	Yes	—
Pressure felt	—	Yes	—	—	Yes	—
Improvements suggested	—	Yes	—	—	Yes	—
No. of beds occupied	22	23	23	24	24	23

*Weekend

Table 4.2 Sister Green. Daily profiles — problems, pressure and improvements. Surgical ward, 20 beds.

	Morning	Morning*	Afternoon	Afternoon*	Evening	Evening
Description of the day	Average Busy	Bad Quiet	Average Busy	Good Average	Good Busy	Average Average
Problems experienced	Yes	—	Yes	—	Yes	—
Pressure felt	—	—	Yes	—	—	—
Improvements suggested	—	—	Yes	—	—	—
No. of beds occupied	16	15	17	15	16	14

*Weekend

and 'adequate senior staff on'. She felt that there had been fewer interruptions, and observation confirmed that fewer activities were initiated by others on this 'quiet' morning. Sister Gold felt that she had been able to spend extra time with the patients, an activity she enjoyed. However, observation showed that in fact she spent considerably less time with patients on this quiet morning — 30 per cent compared with 50 per cent on the busy morning. The discrepancy between perception of time spent with patients and actual time spent may have been related to the fact that on the quiet morning sister felt more 'in control', more organised and better informed. As a result, the pace of work appeared more relaxed and she felt that her time was being used more effectively and enjoyably.

Nursing officer–unit meetings

Sister Gold also experienced pressure on the first evening. One nurse was off sick; there was no staff nurse on; a sisters' meeting earlier in the afternoon 'went on far too long' and delayed her return to the ward. Sister felt anxiously preoccupied with 'all the things to be done and organised': 'when I feel rushed it's easy to make mistakes'. The nursing officer aggravated the situation by arriving 'at the wrong time at the start of the drug round and kept me back for 15 minutes'. When asked about ways in which the evening's work might have been improved, the only suggestion offered was 'one more senior nurse on'. No further remarks were made about the unsuitable timing of the nursing officer's visit or about the expectations surrounding attendance at unit meetings. It seemed that sister felt that she had to be there despite the perceived more urgent need to be in the ward. Minutes of meetings were not available when absent.

Sister Green (Table 4.2)

Too quiet

The 'bad' day which had the lowest total SD score was described, not as a busy day but as a very quiet day. This Sunday morning was 'extra quiet' because the ward was 'well staffed and because patients could do a lot for themselves'. Sister remarked that it was 'not so satisfactory when quiet'. Despite describing the day as 'bad', when asked whether she had any problems she said, 'No . . . but we'd have had more to do if we'd had fewer staff . . . it's crazy.' She seemed to feel that because the usual cry was for more staff, implying that fewer staff could be an improvement seemed a 'crazy' idea. When asked in what way the day could have been improved, no suggestion was offered; she simply remarked that usually 'being better organised' helped but that particular improvement could not apply to a day which was already well organised.

Fluctuating workload

Sister Green felt that peaks and troughs in workload were to be expected in a surgical ward. On the first morning the problem was getting unexpected, unplanned work completed on time. The work was 'under control' until two patients had to be prepared for emergency surgery. Nurses had to leave the ward to accompany patients to theatre and as a result the nursing team became smaller just when the workload increased.

During this time sister became 'irritated' by the 'unprofessional' behaviour of students who started shouting to each other using Christian names, and in the bustle of activity she was too busy to deal with their behaviour promptly. She perceived herself as disapproving (scale score 3), dissatisfied (3) and irritable (3) on the SD scales for the Self with nurses concept, and weak (2) on the Self as sister concept.

Pressure was felt on the first evening when several unplanned technical procedures had to be completed at the same time as the planned work of serving meals. Because there were enough staff on this occasion to complete the work, the temporary pressure was not a problem and sister 'enjoyed' the 'organised, not chaotic busyness'.

Nursing officer – unit meetings

One other difficulty was mentioned on the first afternoon. Sister Green spent 55 minutes out of the ward at a unit meeting with the nursing officer. She felt 'irritated' about the 'repercussions' when away from the ward for a prolonged period. The morning's work had not been completed when sister left for the meeting; the staff nurse was harassed; the other nurses were new to the ward. Sister felt that the meeting was important, but she was uncomfortable out of the ward and wanted to be back quickly to finish off her work and to see how the staff were coping. As a result of the conflict, she felt 'pressure all afternoon'. She felt that the dilemma was her own fault because she had let herself 'get behind with the work in the morning'. Like Sister Gold, Sister Green felt that she ought to be present and that the nursing officer would expect her to attend all meetings. Once again, minutes of meetings were not available when absent.

Table 4.3 Sister Grey. Daily profiles — problems, pressure and improvements. Medical ward, 25 beds

	Morning	Morning*	Afternoon*	Afternoon	Evening	Evening
Description of the day	Average Busy	Average Busy	Good Average	Average Busy	Good Quiet	Bad Busy
Problems experienced	—	—	—	—	—	Yes
Pressure felt	Yes	—	—	Yes	—	Yes
Improvements suggested	Yes	—	—	Yes	—	Yes
No. of beds occupied	22	20	21	24	21	22

*Weekend

MAIN STUDY

Sister Grey (Table 4.3)

The morning, the afternoon and the evening which prompted comments about problems and pressures were each part of a consultants' ward round day.

Routine

On the 'bad' evening which had the lowest total SD score there were more high dependency patients and only two junior nurses on duty: a first year pupil, and a first year student new to the ward. Sister felt under pressure because there was 'a lot to do and think about after the round'. Despite being busy and short staffed, she tried 'to do everything' and got 'annoyed' if tasks were left undone. She felt that other wards used lack of staff as an excuse for omitting work, but remarked, 'I hate it if work is not done . . . I take it as a personal affront.' Despite being aware of priority and changing needs of ill patients, and despite inadequate staffing, sister kept strictly to the usual evening routine and tried to get through all the work by moving more quickly than usual. When discussing ways in which the evening could be improved, the answer to the problem of getting through the heavy workload was 'an extra nurse'. It seemed that when the emphasis was on keeping to routine, staffing and workload fluctuations led to difficulty completing the routine, and this was regarded as a failure and a lowering of standards.

Ward round morning

The events of the ward round morning are described in detail because they led to very great pressure for Sister Grey, and for the author.

Sister Grey worked at a faster pace than all other sisters observed. She had the largest number of brief observed activities and the most fragmentation of activity (Appendix 2). Although this morning was not the busiest observed period in terms of total number of activities recorded, the period from 07.30 hours to 10.30 hours before the ward round involved rapid pursuit of a very fast moving sister and the recording of many brief activities. It was difficult to see and record all that sister did.

Sister Grey made the following remarks about this 'busy' morning:

> We always run like idiots on Thursday. We run every morning but there's a time limit on Thursday. We have to have things ready for the round at 10.30 . . . we work fast . . . never get breaks . . . we have to get their [consultants] sandwiches ready. It's the principle I object to, but it's always been like that.

How did she feel about the time spent with patients?

> Not particularly satisfied . . . can't get time for even a two minute chat with each. Quite frankly, I worry about getting things done today. Their [patients] worries are of secondary importance to getting the sandwiches done. I don't really agree with that but there it is.

How did she feel about the time spent with doctors?

> We have to respect the fact that they have to have a round to see their patients.

How did she feel about the time spent with nurses?

> The ideal is to have one qualified and one student together but on Thursday I pick the fastest workers . . . the auxiliary, she's fast . . . she's been here so long, she knows what to do.

Did she feel under pressure?

> Yes. Right from the start. I come on at 6.30 a.m. on round mornings, 7 a.m. other days. I've got used to it, but my family get mad. . . .

Could she identify any particular problems?

> No . . . not really.

Time targets
As a nurse observer, it was difficult for the author to remain passive and uninvolved in a situation which became more and more fren-

zied and noisy. It seemed that in order to 'get through' the morning's work, all of which had to be done by 10.30, sister set 'objectives' and targets for the staff, that is, time targets — 20 minutes to make all the beds; 10 minutes to get patients back to bed; 15 minutes to get lockers cleaned, case notes and X-rays out. Because the author carried a watch, sister asked for times to be called out, providing a countdown to 10.30. To exhort the nurses into working faster, patients were encouraged to increase the volume of music from radios. As the pace increased, the noise level rose. The nurses had to shout to be heard; linen trolleys knocked against bed-ends and chairs banged; patients started whistling and the author started humming; sister darted back and forth, tidying beds and furnishings; a nurse shouted for some quiet because she could not hear when recording blood pressures.

At 10.33 it became apparent that sister's method of management by time targets was successful. At 10.35 the medical staff arrived to a silent and tidy ward, with all patients in bed and no nurses in sight except sister and myself.

Effects of this pre-round, task-oriented, flurry of activity on some patients became evident: one left the ward temporarily; another remarked that he had thought peace and quiet was needed after a heart attack; a patient in pain asked that the radio on the next locker be turned down but his request was not heard; a high dependency mentally subnormal patient was returned to bed unwashed after being incontinent of urine. It seemed that what Sister Grey described as 'Management by objectives' was a system of timed deadlines for the completion of tasks and this style of management, where the time and the task became the objectives, militated against the provision of individualised patient care.

As the round progressed quietly, many patients fell asleep, and the noise of radios was replaced by loud snoring. The non-participant observer role continued to be difficult, however; as there were no other nurses in the ward area, several patients beckoned to the author for help — for example, to replace a dropped oxygen mask or to ask for a drink of water — and this help was given if the patients were unable to call to sister or ring for a nurse. Although sister was clearly not happy with certain aspects of ward round morning, it is interesting that no specific difficulties were identified or described when she was given the opportunity to talk about problems and ways of improving the day's work.

Sister valued neatness and order, speed and efficiency; she liked to be 'organised' at all times, and the organised–disorganised scale consistently had the maximum SD scale score for every concept. To be 'organised' and ready for 10.30 was a challenge. Yet, sister was aware of disadvantages associated with working at speed, such as having only brief contacts with patients and appearing to be less available to them.

Sister Grey talked on several occasions about sister–consultant relationships, describing consultants as having 'too much power' and making unrealistic demands upon nurses' time. She seemed to feel frustrated by her own lack of power to challenge her medical colleagues. She disapproved of sandwich-making for consultants, and she felt that 10.30 a.m. was an unrealistic time by which to have all the work done; yet the ward round pattern of activity and the sandwich-making continued. There was no indication whether the consultants were aware of or would have approved of the pre-round ward activity. The only solutions to the pressures felt on the morning of the consultants' round were, in the sister's opinion, 'to start the round later' or 'to be better staffed'.

Semantic differential scores for the ward round morning confirmed Sister Grey's difficulties (Table 4.4).

Table 4.4 Sister Grey. Semantic differential scale scores on ward round morning

	Self with doctors	Self with patients	Self with nurses	Self as sister
Approving–disapproving	3	5	4	4
Organised–disorganised	7	7	7	7
Active–passive	1	7	5	7
Influential–uninfluential	1	4	5	7
Calm–irritable	7	7	5	5
Attentive–inattentive	6	5	3	6
Beneficial–harmful	5	5	6	7
Sociable–unsociable	4	7	3	7
Strong–weak	3	4	6	4
Satisfied–dissatisfied	3	5	5	7
Total concept score	40	56	49	59

Maximum scale score = 7

Although active, satisfied and influential on the whole, Sister Grey felt passive, uninfluential, less satisfied, less strong and less approving of self when working with the doctors. The concept Self with doctors had the lowest total concept score on each day.

Sister Brown (Table 4.5)
Sister Brown consistently gave high scores on all the SD scales throughout the study. The high ratings, however, did seem to reflect her feelings at the time and her comments showed that she was

Table 4.5 Sister Brown. Daily profiles — problems, pressure and improvements. Medical ward, 25 beds

	Morning	Morning*	Afternoon	Afternoon*	Evening	Evening
Description of the day	Good Quiet	Good Quiet	Good Quiet	Good Quiet	Average Busy	Average Quiet
Problems experienced	Yes	—	—	—	—	—
Pressure felt	—	—	—	—	Yes	—
Improvements suggested	—	—	—	—	—	—
No. of beds occupied	22	21	21	15	23	20

*Weekend

Table 4.6 Sister White. Daily profiles — problems, pressure and improvements. Medical ward, 25 beds

	Morning*	Morning	Afternoon	Afternoon*	Evening	Evening
Description of the day	Good Quiet	Average Average	Good Quiet	Average Busy	Good Average	Good Busy
Problems experienced	—	Yes	—	—	—	Yes
Pressure felt	—	—	—	Yes	—	Yes
Improvements suggested	—	—	—	—	—	—
No. of beds occupied	18	18	18	18	21	20

*Weekend

experiencing fewer problems and was less worried about them than the other sisters. She often remarked about her enjoyment of the job and made fewer critical remarks than her colleagues about the sister's role.

Negative scores were given on only one morning for the Self with patients concept. On this morning, sister accompanied the consultants for one and a half hours on their ward round and felt passive and uninfluential with patients. The morning was described as 'very good' because there were 'plenty staff', work was done 'at a leisurely pace', and 'the atmosphere at the round was relaxed and friendly'.

The only problem identified concerned a clerical error in the records department. An ambulance failed to arrive, and sister had to find time to make alternative arrangements and explain to the patient the reason for the delay.

The optimum pace of work

During 'good', 'quiet', 'well staffed' periods, Sister Brown enjoyed being able to give extra time to aspects of her work she considered important, such as, 'becoming involved with patients', and 'working with each nurse'. She felt, however, that the ward could be too quiet. On the afternoon when there were only 15 patients, and few acutely ill, she remarked that it would have been good for all the staff to 'have a patient admitted'. She felt that there was an optimum pace of work for nurses; the challenge of the acutely ill admission 'perked the nurses up' and 'made a difference to ward atmosphere'. A slack pace of work was not necessarily desirable.

On the evening rated 'busy', the pace of work was much faster. During this period there were 23 patients including one whose condition deteriorated rapidly, requiring preparation for emergency surgery. There were only two nurses on duty with sister, one of whom did not know the ward, but Sister Brown remarked that she enjoyed being 'extra busy' and 'coped with it all'. She felt that spending time 'working with nurses individually' could be 'beneficial to sister and nurse'; it allowed her to 'explain things' to the nurse and 'answer the nurse's questions'. The suggested improvement was to have one extra nurse.

Sister White (Table 4.6)

Sister White described the patient care workload during the study as lighter than usual. She felt that staffing levels were adequate or more than adequate on all but one day.

A 'good' day for Sister White was one with 'no admissions', 'not too many very ill patients' and with 'plenty of staff who knew the ward routine' and could do work for her. She enjoyed a day when she did not have to rush anyone and she felt that her job was 'just to keep an eye on things'.

The first problem was the arrival, on ward round morning, of two doctors new to the ward. Sister White felt she had to spend extra time with them 'to tell them the routine'. Without this extra work, she said that 'there would have been very little to do' because there were 'so many staff on'.

The second problem, on an evening, was being 'one nurse short' and having a first year student, who had never been in the ward, sent to help. The suggested improvement was to have a nurse sent who already knew the ward routine.

Nursing officer – unit meetings
The other suggested improvement concerned unit meetings. The nursing officer had given sister only one hour's notice to attend a unit meeting one afternoon when there was much extra detailed work to be done after the morning ward round. Sister was willing to delegate work, but had little time to arrange this. She felt that dates and times of meetings should be decided in advance so that work could be planned to take into account a lengthy period away from the ward, and she suggested that some days such as ward round days just were not suitable for meetings.

Sister Black (Table 4.7)
During the study, Sister Black described the ward as 'unusually quiet', 'like a holiday'. Just before Christmas, waiting lists had been reduced and one theatre had closed. On two occasions there were only seven and nine patients in the ward.

Too quiet
The highest and the lowest SD scores occurred on days described as 'good' and 'quiet'. On each occasion sister had three nurses on duty including a staff nurse, but on the high score morning there were 19 patients, and on the low score evening only seven patients. Sister Black disliked being too quiet. The evening was 'good' because the staff had no trouble getting through the little work there was, but sister remarked, 'I just haven't anything to do.' She felt that quiet spells were 'more tiring' than busy spells: when quiet, 'wee things get forgotten'; when busy, she felt able to 'concentrate better' because she had to 'make an effort' to get on with work. Even on the morning with 19 patients, sister would have preferred 'more to do'.

Table 4.7 Sister Black. Daily profiles — problems, pressure and improvements. Surgical ward, 26 beds

	Morning	Morning*	Afternoon	Afternoon*	Evening	Evening
Description of the day	Good Quiet	Good Quiet	Good Quiet	Average Quiet	Average Busy	Good Quiet
Problems experienced	—	—	—	Yes	—	—
Pressure felt	—	Yes	—	—	Yes	—
Improvements suggested	—	—	—	—	—	—
No. of beds occupied	19	9	20	14	20	7

*Weekend

Table 4.8 Sister Pink. Daily profiles — problems, pressure and improvements. Surgical ward, 26 beds

	Morning	Morning*	Afternoon	Afternoon*	Evening	Evening
Description of the day	Average Average	Good Busy	Good Quiet	Good Quiet	Good Average	Good Quiet
Problems experienced	Yes	—	—	Yes	Yes	—
Pressure felt	Yes	—	Yes	Yes	Yes	—
Improvements suggested	—	—	—	—	—	—
No. of beds occupied	20	24	17	12	15	13

*Weekend

During the quiet evening, sister 'spent a lot more time in the duty room' preparing duty rotas, a job usually done at home but selected on this occasion in preference to spending time with nurses or patients. 'If I'd wanted to, I could have spent more time with them . . .' Despite disliking being quiet, no problem was identified or improvement suggested: 'All that needed to be done was done.' SD scores for the concept Self as sister for the quiet evening showed that although Sister Black felt calm (7), sociable (7), beneficial (6) and organised (5), she also felt passive (1), uninfluential (1), inattentive (2) and weak (2).

When trying to identify the elements in a 'good' day, Sister Black suggested that there was an ideal amount of work and level of staffing which kept her 'busy' but not 'frantic', which provided stimulation and forced her to think, and allowed time for talking with patients: 'nursing patients', rather than simply doing procedures — 'nursing drips'.

The two suggested improvements were 'more to do' when quiet, and 'another nurse' when busy.

Supplies policy

The only problem concerned a recent decision to stop supplying string to tie laundry bags because of the expense of string. Bandages were being used instead. Supplies department then questioned the excessive ordering of expensive bandages. Sister Black felt irritated by 'senseless economies' and by the lack of discussion and failure to agree on a policy for the matter.

Sister Pink (Table 4.8)

During January the ward was still felt to be 'quiet' despite a return to full theatre lists and waiting list admissions. On two occasions there were only 12 and 13 patients.

Too quiet

Sister Pink, the junior sister, shared her senior colleague's feelings about being 'quiet'. After a quiet afternoon she remarked that she 'couldn't work up any enthusiasm', 'felt lazy', 'couldn't be bothered doing the little there was to do'. She felt that she was 'wasting' her time; 'the only pressure I felt today was from sitting so long'. She remarked, 'We moan if we're busy but we enjoy it better.' The suggested improvements were 'a bit more work'.

During the quieter afternoon when there were only 12 patients, and 10 nurses on duty including the two sisters, Sister Pink had no contact with two first year students; she spent 8 minutes and 4 minutes respectively with the other two first year students, 13 minutes and 3 minutes with the auxiliaries, and 100 minutes with her senior colleague Sister Black. During this afternoon, when feeling less enthusiastic, sister did not go out into the patient area to talk to visitors despite having enough time to do so and despite considering this an important part of her work.

Sister felt pressure on two occasions: first, when she had difficulty finding time to complete a supplies order in addition to routine work; and second, when two consultants arrived unexpectedly and wanted to discuss a patient care problem with sister while she was busy doing a patient's dressing. As a result, a student nurse had to complete the dressing unsupervised, and work had to be quickly reallocated. Sister felt that she should always be 'free to organise' ward work rather than be involved in it directly.

SUMMARY

Just over half (23) of the 42 observed periods were described as good and only three as bad. In terms of perceived pressure of work, there were more periods described as quiet (19) than busy (15). Four sisters felt at some point during the study that they had too little to do and both busy and quiet periods were considered bad.

Problems were identified on eight of the 42 observed periods and the solutions suggested tended to be simple and short term. Certain problems which clearly existed were not stated, however, usually because the sisters felt that nothing could be done about those problems rather than because they failed to 'see' or understand them.

The following problem areas were identified:

1. Lack of control over workload and nurse staffing levels, and inability to provide the right number of nurses with the levels of skills required to meet fluctuating patient care demands; there could be too many or too few nurses.

2. Lack of suitably qualified or sufficiently competent staff to whom sister's work could be safely delegated in her absence; when this occurred, sisters disliked leaving the ward or being out of the ward for long periods.

3. Information overload when trying to assimilate quickly large amounts of rapidly changing information, particularly when admitting and discharging patients, on ward round days, or after days off. The sisters suggested that the frequency and level of this problem was influenced by several interrelated factors: the number of patients, the number of consultants, the frequency of doctor's ward rounds,

and the admission and discharge policies of the ward.

4. Being too quiet and having too little to do. It was suggested that there was an optimum pace and amount of work which was stimulating and satisfying. Levels above and below the optimum were tiring and disliked.

5. Having difficulty completing work and providing individualised care when adhering to work routines based on time targets.

6. Inability to challenge medically sanctioned routine and policy, and the perception of doctors as more powerful than nurses.

7. Filling perceived gaps in the services of other professionals or other departments in the interests of prompt, safe patient care.

8. Unit meetings: nursing officers failed to provide adequate notice of meetings and held them at unsuitable times. Conflict existed between the self-expectation of the sister that she ought to go and the perceived, if not the actual, expectation of the nursing officer that the sister must go to unit meetings.

9. Policies for the ordering and provision of certain ward supplies were unclear.

The perception of the day as good or bad largely depended upon whether or not the sister felt 'in control' of what was going on, and the feeling of being 'in control' seemed to be influenced mainly by the absence or presence of the first three problem areas.

5

Twenty-five problems

Did the nine sisters agree about which problems were most worrying? A first glance at the rankings suggested little agreement. Table 5.1 shows that 11 statements were ranked first or second as the greatest problems, 10 statements were ranked twenty-fourth or twenty-fifth as the least problems and the range of rank positions for some statements was very wide. 'Doing basic nursing care' was ranked first by one sister and twenty-fifth by another.

Looking only at the extremes of range, however, is misleading. For example, 'Being interrupted so often' has a range of rank order positions from 1 to 23, but eight of the nine sisters ranked it between 1 and 8 and only the ninth sister ranked it as 23.

The rankings and ratings of each sister for every statement are shown in Appendix 3.

To measure the degree of agreement between the sisters in their independent ranking of the 25 statements Kendall's coefficient of concordance was used (Siegel 1956). A statistically significant result was obtained indicating a strong probability ($P < 0.001$) that the agreement found was greater than could have been expected to have occurred by chance.

The relationship between the rankings of pairs of sisters was also examined, using Spearman's rank order correlation coefficient (Siegel 1956). Comparisons were made between senior sisters, junior sisters, two sisters in the same ward, most experienced sisters, least experienced sisters, medical sisters and surgical sisters. A number of strongly positive relationships were found but they did not seem to be associated with these pairing criteria and it was difficult to account for the similarities between the sisters.

The correlations did suggest, however, that one sister was different. When Sister White's rankings were paired with those of all other sisters, negative or only weakly positive correlations were obtained (Appendix 4). Sister White's interview comments will show that she did differ from her colleagues in many ways.

From the remarks about each statement which follow, it will be

Table 5.1 Problem statements: range of rank positions and the overall rank order for each statement

	Rank order*	Range of rank positions
Having enough contact with the patients	1	1–14
Finding time to talk with patients in a leisurely way	2	2–10
Being interrupted so often	3.5	1–23
Teaching the student nurses	3.5	2–16
Having enough contact with the student nurses	5	1–17
Meeting the demands of so many people	6	3–17
Being available to everyone while on duty	7	4–20
Having too much to do each day	8.5	1–18
Finding out whether the work is being done	8.5	3–20
Doing basic nursing care	10	1–25
Getting the nursing officer to understand the ward	11	1–20
Feeling tired	12	2–25
Keeping up to date with new trends	13.5	3–24
Disagreeing with a doctor's instructions for a patient	13.5	2–23
Friction between staff	15	6–25
Doing things that are not part of my job	16	2–23
Considering myself as a manager	17.5	7–24
Getting the staff nurses to understand the ward sister's role	17.5	8–23
Not having enough time to myself while on duty	19	9–25
Finding someone to turn to when I need help	20	9–24
Making changes in the ward	21	10–22
Getting the doctors to listen to my point of view	22	10–22
Feeling isolated from other ward sisters	23	10–25
Doing ward work in off-duty time	24	10–25
Understanding my job responsibilities	25	14–25

*Based on rank totals obtained by adding the nine sisters' scores (Appendix 3).

seen that there were many reasons why the sisters did, or did not, feel concerned about various parts of their work.

Predictably, those aspects of work considered most important, such as contact with patients and learners, were the ones which received highest ratings and rankings and caused the sisters most worry.

When statements were given low ratings and rankings, however, it did not necessarily mean that those problems did not exist or that the aspects of work referred to in the statement were less important. Low rankings were given: first, because a problem had been resolved; second, because a problem was being tackled successfully; third, because other problems were more pressing; fourth, because the sister simply did not feel worried about the problem even

although it existed; fifth, because the sister felt nothing could be
done to solve the problem and was resigned to living with it.

SISTER AND THE PATIENTS

The two problem statements concerning contact with patients were
ranked first and second overall. 'Having enough contact with
patients' and 'Finding time to talk with patients in a leisurely
way' worried considerably eight of the nine sisters.

The sisters' comments showed different degrees of understanding of the professional skills used when in contact with patients.

Contact was interpreted in several ways:

Sitting or standing at the bedside talking with a patient
Giving direct patient care, referred to as 'doing basic care' or
'actively nursing'
Doing a sister's round, systematically visiting each patient
Simply being present in the same area as patients, able to see and
be seen by them.

Why was contact important? It was a means of assessing the needs
of patients and it formed the basis of care planning. It required
skilled observation and interviewing.

> If you don't have time to sit down and talk to the patients, you
> cannot find out all the little niggles and worries, and then you
> can't communicate to the students properly, you can't teach
> them properly. I feel that you've got to know your patient in-
> side out before you can plan care, teach the students and make
> some sort of logical sense out of the patient care plan.
>
> Sister Blue

Contact was also important for establishing and maintaining 'good
relationships'. Meeting sister was regarded as an essential courtesy
for a newly admitted patient, and being able to see or talk to the
person in charge was thought to give 'confidence' and 'security'.

> They are guests in your ward and you feel that at some point in
> the day you ought to give them your undivided attention. You
> want to ensure that they realise you are the ward sister and un-
> less you go round to chat with them they can't get to know
> you.
>
> Sister Red

It was suggested that talking with patients 'in a leisurely way'
could mean 'gossip and idle chat'; but it was also interpreted as

skilled, relaxed communication which could lead to 'meaningful conversation out of which you can obtain information discreetly'.

Sister Pink, the least experienced sister, seemed less clear about her assessment role in patient care and about her contribution towards building up sister – patient relationships:

> There are a lot who would not want to talk to you. They like to keep themselves to themselves.... I often feel that the healthier ones don't really want to have that much contact with the sister. They feel that the sister is the boss and they prefer talking to the junior nurses. They will tell them more....

Finding time for contact

Patient contact could be time consuming. Sometimes contacts were brief, lasting only 'a couple of minutes', but there were occasions when longer periods were needed. It seemed that contact with every patient was an important objective but sometimes particular patients required more attention; Sister Red's simple arithmetic highlighted the difficulty of finding time for everyone:

> I have 58 patients. If you devoted one minute to every patient there's your hour up — uninterrupted. You'll come upon a patient who has real problems and you feel you have to sit on the edge of the bed and perhaps devote 15 to 20 minutes. When you feel they must be allowed to open up, that's the difficulty.

Spending long periods of time with patients could be uncomfortable because of the ever-present subjective pressure 'to get on with the work'. Also, it was difficult to concentrate during prolonged contact, because of overt and covert interruptions; that is, interruptions by other people and interruptions of thought within the sister's 'buzzing mind'. The latter type of interruption was described by Sister Red as 'occult interruption' and both kinds of interruption could prevent a sister from feeling that she was giving her undivided attention to a patient.

> It's not always easy to find time just to chat with patients and if you have time maybe your mind is so full of other things. You just can't settle down, and the interruptions come. There are times when I think I'd just love to spend a whole morning going round talking with them all, getting beneath the superficial level. So often you don't really meet their need at the time, for example, patients who come in so worried before operations.
>
> Sister Green

Some sisters did realise that pace of work and pressure varied. They were not always busy and there could be 'a quiet weekend' or 'lots of time' for contact with patients. But observation and the comments of some sisters revealed that available time was not always used constructively; it was not necessarily *lack* of time which limited contact with patients.

Speed of work and control over contact

Several sisters felt that when they were busy and working at speed, some patients could be missed altogether or addressed hurriedly and others who might want to approach them would hesitate because sisters always seemed to be moving so fast. Sister Black remarked:

> You are rushing them all the time. Wee things that are important to them they want to ask you, but they think that the sister is so busy and don't bother.

Sister Gold made morning and evening rounds to see and be seen by her patients in the hope that visibility would equal availability. She had discovered, however, that merely being visible and available did not guarantee adequate contact or effective communication:

> I've got to make a genuine effort to go round morning and evening and hope that the patients will realise that I have time then to talk to them. They feel they mustn't delay you too long. If you don't spend long enough, you don't know how they've interpreted what you've said. Many a time I've found patients who've misinterpreted what I'd told them. Today I had a patient who is to have a fasting blood sugar done and obviously has a dread of needles. Three or four times in the passing he asked, 'Is it only blood I'm to have taken, I'm not to have a sternal marrow?' You begin to wonder what else is going round in his mind.

Sister Grey's dilemma was particularly acute. She chose to work at a fast pace not only to help get through the work but also to control interruptions by being seen to be busy. She knew that making herself less available and approachable created problems, and she felt uneasy when prolonged patient contact became necessary:

> We don't really help by running past them and doing things as fast as we can instead of trying to win over their confidence.

The feeling of being in control of the use of one's own time appeared to be crucial. Patient contact was welcomed but it seemed that the sisters preferred to initiate the contact themselves. Patient-initiated contact could hold sister back; by being available she risked being detained, interrupted or sidetracked. Sister Red commented:

> You go to see the patient, the patient says, 'Ah, Sister, now's my opportunity!' And that leads on to more conversation that is nothing to do with the pressure area you were originally considering. You want the contact with the patient, but at a time that suits you and you want just the right degree of contact.

Assessment of patients — expert versus novice

Sister Red, the most experienced sister, outlined another dilemma. On the one hand, a sister could feel that she was saving time and could feel more comfortable seeing a patient herself to make an 'expert' assessment. On the other hand, she would have to allow less experienced staff to practise and develop their own assessment and reporting skills.

> This feeling within the ward sister that she wants to see the patient herself, or see the bleeding, the pallor, the pressure area, the state of the patient's mouth . . . it goes back to trusting the staff; this is a frustration, that you are dependent on second-hand information. You've to keep saying to the nurse, 'What exactly do you mean? How red is red? Is the skin actually broken?' And, 'Is it blistered?' 'Does it need a dressing?' And so it goes on. In fact you might have been quicker seeing the patient yourself.

Ward layout

Ward 'geography' was thought to influence patient contact. It was felt that sisters used more energy 'keeping an eye' on patients in small rooms, whereas in a Nightingale ward a sister could observe patients and be observed more easily. Sister Blue had a divided ward:

> Because of the pressures of the day and the geography of the ward, you can get through a day seeing very little of the patients on an individual basis. If you had a Nightingale ward the patients would at least see you functioning . . . [in my ward] they can go for a long time without seeing the sister, and actual time to just sit down and talk to them is at a premium.

Observation

The amount of time spent by the sisters in direct contact with patients was calculated. Table 5.2 shows the number of observations and the percentage of time spent by each sister in patient-centred activities throughout the ward, both at bedsides and in other areas such as treatment rooms and bathrooms. The activities included observing and talking with patients, checking charts, giving drugs, carrying out technical procedures and providing basic care, bathing, making beds and attending to comfort and nutrition.

Table 5.2 Sister–patient contact. Number of observations and time spent in patient-centred activities

Sister	Number of observations	Number of minutes	Percentage of time
Gold	315	407	25
Green	343	426	26
Grey	485	500	30
Brown	392	453	27
White	275	284	17
Black	391	392	23
Pink	400	437	26

All except Sister White spent at least 23 per cent of their time on patient-centred work, the range being from 17 to 30 per cent. It can be seen from the table, however, that these considerable percentages of time represented a large number of observations many of which were very brief.

Sister White, who spent the least time with patients, 17 per cent, felt that she had enough contact and did not wish more. Her comments suggested that she had a more limited view of the patient assessment and support functions of her role:

> I think that I have enough contact . . . I just don't want any more than I have. I would like sometimes to talk with them more — just general talk, I do not mean about their condition — for example, to find out what life was like years ago. . . . Sometimes you do not have the time and you have an interesting patient, or lots of time and nobody very interesting to talk to.

Doing basic nursing care

Sister Gold's comment that 'basic nursing care is nursing' seemed to sum up the sisters' feelings. The statement 'Doing basic nursing care' was ranked tenth overall but the extent to which the sisters were worried about this aspect of their work varied considerably. One sister ranked it first as her greatest worry, another ranked it last as her least worry.

The term basic nursing care was interpreted as 'the practical work', bed making, bed bathing, attending to the hair, the mouth, the skin and the nails. It meant being 'close' to patients and dealing with the 'little details' of nursing.

Providing direct patient care was 'enjoyable' and helped 'to keep up morale'. It gave opportunities for assessing patients and for keeping an eye on learners and the standards of care given.

> Basically I enjoy this. I really like to get stuck in and do the nails and the hair. If you get a new student, and if you can get her into good basic nursing care, not only do you set her off on the right road but there's a terrific sense of satisfaction out of it.
>
> Sister Blue

> You see them bed bathing but they never think to comb hair ... somebody with a dry mouth, they never think to give oral hygiene or clean their teeth. You have really got to be watching them all the time. I think standards have fallen. We have not got a lot of senior staff and it is just impossible for one person to watch everything that is going on. If you have got the time, you can go with the student nurses and show them how to do it properly. I think some of them don't really care that much. Some of them come into the ward looking as if they haven't combed their hair themselves.
>
> Sister Pink

Sister Pink was also unhappy about the greater interest in 'high status technical care' at the expense of 'basic care' and her colleague in the same ward, Sister Black, remarked:

> They seem to think that if they can give an injection and do a blood pressure they are great. ... It's difficult getting them to realise that washing a patient, cleaning his mouth is just as important. ... They tend to forget that it's a person they are nursing.

The main difficulty for the sisters seemed to be finding time for giving care because of the demands of other work, particularly 'administration'. Lack of time for giving basic care meant reduced job satisfaction, and less opportunity to teach and assess learners' clinical expertise. It also contributed to the uncomfortable feeling of not knowing what was happening to patients.

Sister Gold remarked:

> Basic nursing care is nursing. By the time you get to be ward sister you have lost that opportunity which I regret deeply. I sometimes come away feeling at the end of the day that because all I've done is sit and do administrative work or organise things I haven't actually done nursing.

Some sisters realised that their role in the nursing team had to be different from that of staff nurses and learners. The transition from learner to staff nurse to sister could mean a reduction in time spent in 'real nursing', giving care, and an increase in the time spent organising the team to give the care.

> It's the ward sister's role that you get further away from the patients. Maybe it's no worse than being a nursing officer. We are trained to be nurses; nursing is the practical work and it's very hard to divorce yourself from that.

> Sister Green

Sister Blue felt that learning to differentiate her role from others in the team and to cope with the complex blend of clinical, teaching and administrative responsibilities was extremely difficult. It needed skilled management:

> I don't have nearly enough time to work with the new students. You find that they'll do a blanket bath. If you're lucky they'll do the hair. They're quite likely to forget about the mouth wash. They probably won't look at the nails and between the toes. They won't observe the condition of the skin; they are not really *observing* . . . they've got to be taught, and unless you can get in and work with them you can't point these things out. It's the little details . . . this worries me a lot. You are just torn between your administrative duties and your practical, teaching duties . . . there are so many other things to be dealt with. . . . Perhaps I should have put understanding management further up, but I just don't know how to manage that ward any differently and this is where a really good unit nursing officer might be able to point something out.

Sister Blue understood that to some extent she had to stand back from direct care in order to coordinate and effectively 'manage' the nursing. She was clear about her role responsibilities as manager, but felt that she lacked adequate support and gave this problem maximum rating. In contrast there were two sisters who seemed less clear about being managers of the nursing team. They both considered involvement in basic care as the least of their worries and gave the problem lowest rating.

> I like to try to do basic nursing care. Some sisters are quite happy to sit in the duty room and delegate but I couldn't do that.
>
> Sister Black

> That's the least of my worries because I enjoy giving basic nursing care. . . . I'd hate to lose touch. I'd hate to sit in the office and issue orders.
>
> Sister White

Sister Red, the most experienced sister, summed up the dilemma in her 'sheer joy of nursing' remark. Over the years she had learned that having less time for the most enjoyable part of nursing was regrettable but inevitable, and she had come to terms with the dilemma. The fact that she was less worried about this problem at the time of the study was probably due not only to experience and being clear about her role responsibilities, but also feeling that she was well supported by her nursing officer, by her clinical teacher and by the other sister in the ward:

> I don't suppose this really worries me. We all like to do a procedure on our own without someone to teach, without feeling you are being watched, just for the sheer joy of nursing. We are all in the job for that reason. It's an inevitable part of sistering that you do have to allow others to do an awful lot of the basic nursing care. It just depends how well organised you are yourself how much time you can get involved in basic nursing care. But there's no doubt about it that now and again you have to do a wee bit of it just to keep your own morale up.

Finding out about work
The statement 'Finding out whether the work is being done' was in tied rank position of 8.5 overall.

The four sisters who were worried about this problem and who gave it high rating and ranking showed that finding out about work is a complex issue related to several factors in the sister's management of her nursing team; it is related, to the way in which work is prescribed, to the system of supervising and assessing the work of learners and to the system of reporting back and exacting accountability for work done.

None of the seven who were observed seemed to have a system which gave nurses clear accountability for reporting back verbally or in writing about their work. The sisters checked personally whether work had been done, or they asked nurses about their work at report times and as they moved round the ward. The nurses seldom volunteered information even at reports and the sisters themselves took responsibility for writing up the Kardex about each patient's care.

Sister Blue, who was interviewed but not observed, was the only sister who was able to describe clearly a daily nursing management cycle similar to that outlined by Pembrey (1980): that is, she claimed to carry out a nursing round of patients, followed by a full report with prescription and delegation of work to a group of nurses responsible for a group of patients, and finally she received accountability reports from nurses about each patient. Despite having this system, Sister Blue still experienced difficulties with finding out about work; and it was Sister Blue who gave the highest rating and ranking to this problem statement. For example, she had doubts not only about whether all prescribed work was done, but also about whether the work had been done to an acceptable standard. She felt that adequate supervision of learners was essential; however, if there were too few or no staff nurses on duty with her, then as sister she had to be actively involved in checking personally the amount and standard of work done:

> You can write up work in the nursing care plan; you can allocate a nurse to do it; but you can't be certain that it's being done. The girls are very honest and usually admit if they haven't done it, but there's always the odd one who's likely to pull the wool over your eyes. She can go off down to the other end of the ward where you can't see her and you don't know *how* she has done it . . . standard is pretty important.

Sister Blue encouraged learners to document their own work but that also posed difficulties because considerable amounts of time had to be spent teaching the learners how to write their own reports accurately:

> Another thing is the risk you take getting them to write their own reports because obviously they're learning. In the nursing Kardex report they write down what they've done but some are too general and not concise and relevant enough.

In contrast, other sisters who 'checked up' to find out about work seemed much less aware of the personal accountability of each learner to report back:

> If I ask the nurses to do something, I find it difficult to leave them. As a new ward sister, I'd go into the duty room and shut the door and I'd be out in two seconds checking them, but I'm getting better at this. I give them time to do it and then go in and check that they have done it. I couldn't sit in the duty room all day; I have to be checking that they've done it.
>
> Sister Black

> I don't find that too bad because I have got into the habit of checking everything after it is done. . . . it depends on the seniority of the nurse . . . as they get more senior you can rely on them.
>
> Sister Pink

The extent to which the sister had 'trust' in a nurse's competence influenced the need to 'check up' on performance. Sister Brown was particularly anxious about the abilities of learners new to the ward. However, she felt secure once staff had the ward 'routine off pat' and she seemed to assume that prescribed work was done if the nurses got through the routine:

> When you have a new lot of students and pupils to the ward, they do not know your routine, they are a wee bit apprehensive, they do not know the patients . . . you have really got to keep an eye on them. My permanent staff, I know their abilities, I know they have their routine off pat and they can get on with it.

Fluctuations in numbers and grades of nurses in the team from day to day influenced the ways in which sisters found out about work done. When staff nurses were on duty, it was felt that they could be relied on to report back; but students had to be checked up on. A sister would relax if she had on duty with her a staff nurse who had enough experience and skill in assessment to respond to changing needs of patients, needs which would have to be met outwith routine. Student nurses, however, would lack experience and skill to adapt routine flexibly to meet changing needs. In these circumstances a sister would want to check that matters which she considered 'priorities' were being dealt with.

> In the morning you probably have a staff nurse or a senior nurse who can report to you accurately and punctually, but in

the evening you may well be on with just student nurses. The students may not appreciate the priorities.

Sister Brown

The final two remarks draw together the difficulties with finding out about work, Sister Red characteristically considering the problem from a number of viewpoints and Sister Green neatly summing it up as a matter requiring 'organisation'.

There's quite a lot in that statement really . . . checking that it's being done, that it's being done properly, checking in such a way that you are not going to upset the people who've done it, having enough time to find out . . . it's knowing first and foremost whether you can trust the staff that you've allocated to a certain job. The less you know a person, the less you trust them and the more you feel you've got to find out whether they are doing the work properly.

Sister Red

I suppose it comes down to organising yourself and your work and making sure that the nurses come and report back.

Sister Green

SISTER AND THE LEARNERS

The sisters gave similar rankings and ratings to the two statements about learners. 'Teaching the student nurses' was in tied rank position of 3.5 overall and 'Having enough contact with the student nurses' was ranked fifth overall. The term student was used for student and pupil nurses, as both groups of learners were referred to as 'the students' by the sisters.

Why was contact with learners felt to be so important? Contact was needed to establish good 'relationships' and to 'get to know' the students. Establishing a good relationship was regarded as part of the wider objective of fostering a good ward atmosphere based on free communication between staff. Getting to know the student included not only assessment of professional competence but also learning about the nurse 'as a person'. For example, it was important to be sensitive to problems with home and family life which might be worrying a learner and affecting her performance at work. Sister Gold remarked:

I don't often have the chance to work with them and therefore I don't get the little things, like home life, that may be relevant. This strongly bothers me considering I am supposed to be training them. If I had more time, I feel I would get to know them much better and therefore have a better understanding of them as people, and also know more of what they require to learn.

As Sister Gold indicated, contact with students was also important in relation to a sister's teaching function; teaching, training, identifying learning needs and relating practice to theory were all mentioned as being part of sister's work.

The problems experienced by the sisters in getting contact with learners and in using it effectively were lack of time, having several priorities competing for their time, and the status barrier.

Lack of time for contact

During observation, each nurse in every grade in the ward team was given a personal code. It was therefore possible to see how often and for how long each nurse had direct contact with her sister, working or simply talking together.

Observation showed that the sisters often spent very small amounts of time with learners and that the grade which spent least time with the sister was the first year student nurse.

In the pilot study wards several nurses had very little contact with Sisters Gold and Green, for example, as little as one minute for a first year student nurse during a five and a half hour evening period. First year students and pupils tended to have less contact with their sister than second or third year students and most contacts were brief.

In the first main study ward, pupil nurses spent more time with Sister Grey than student nurses and, of all learners, pupils and students, the first year student spent least time with sister. One evening, Sister Grey had only two junior nurses on duty with her: a first year student who had started working in the ward that day, and a first year pupil nurse. Only 7 per cent of the student's time was spent with sister compared with 27 per cent of the pupil's. Both nurses needed close supervision and teaching, especially the student new to the ward. But on this busy evening when sister was short of staff, in order to get the work done, she chose the pupil nurse who was familiar with ward routine to accompany her to give patient care. The student nurse had to work alone and unsupervised.

When under pressure Sister Grey worked with the nurse who knew the ward best and who could move at speed; in this instance, the pupil nurse. On other occasions she chose a senior student rather than a junior student, or even an auxiliary in preference to any grade of student, possibly because the two auxiliaries, who had worked seven years and four years respectively in this ward, were trusted, considered competent and could work at Sister Grey's hectic pace.

When pressure dropped and staffing improved, Sister Grey did give time to the least experienced students and pupils, but even in the quieter periods the student learner had less time with sister than the pupil. Busy or quiet, the student became the loser in the contact stakes.

In the second and third main study wards, the findings were similar. Contacts were brief, except at ward reports, and often the junior learners spent as little as 1 or 2 per cent of their time with sister.

The sisters said they wanted contact with students to help them feel that they were participating fully in the ward team, to teach them, to assess their performance and to identify their work difficulties.

The information from observing the sisters, similar to the findings in Lelean's (1973) study, did suggest that the sisters who were worried about contact did have grounds for concern about lack of time with students. Their concern was diffuse, however, and not related to junior learners in particular. But it is important to note that not all sisters were worried about lack of contact; one of the less experienced sisters, Sister White, felt that she had enough contact with learners and did not wish more.

Competing priorities

Clinical, teaching and administrative responsibilities all made demands on time and some sisters did not feel they could give teaching enough attention because of the pressure of other work. Sister Green pointed out the dilemma of having to balance the demands of administration against the wish to spend time to 'work with' the students. She felt that this contributed to the problem of having only a superficial picture of the students' capabilities:

> So often we just don't get to know the students . . . you only get a very superficial picture of what they are doing in the ward. Because of all the management and administrative things, you don't actually get a chance to work with them.

Status barrier

Sister Black, Sister White and Sister Pink talked of difficulties in establishing comfortable working relationships with learners.

Sister Black saw the problem as having to balance a disciplined approach with a friendly approach. Throughout her six years as sister she had been uncertain about handling work relationships, and she attributed her insecurity to 'lack of confidence' in her teaching ability and to her 'personality':

> I just don't know how friendly I should get with them ... in the past the nurses have said that I am very strict and not really interested in them as people. ... I feel that you still have to have a certain amount of discipline in the ward and I some-times just don't feel that I can get a happy balance, I tend to be a bit strict rather than lenient with them.

Sister White was sure that status did block communication from student to sister but she suggested that the barrier was necessary; and she did not want more contact with learners:

> Once you become a ward sister then there is a certain barrier. ... There are certain things they will tell you and certain things they will not tell you. ... The barrier has to be there otherwise you do not run your ward. I think I get enough contact as it is ... I don't think I would want any more contact.

Sister Pink's remark about students being 'scared' of a sister seemed to be related to the fact that she had not been in her junior sister post for very long; at the time of the study she still identified more with the staff nurse role than with the sister role:

> Student nurses go to a staff nurse before they come to a sister. The sister is too far away from them. I suppose they are a bit scared of you. If they have someone (a staff nurse) in between to go to, then I find out more about the student nurses.

Teaching
Teaching worried all the sisters and it was the most frequently mentioned reason for needing contact with learners. The problems found were lack of time for teaching, uncertainty about what to teach and how to teach, lack of confidence in teaching ability, lack of expert specialist help and difficulty assessing the learning needs and performance of students.

Several types of teaching were identified: teaching by example, formal tutorials and lectures.

Teaching by example
Teaching by example was regarded as possible, desirable and enjoy-

able. It was possible, using brief contacts with students in patient areas, contacts which might last for only a few minutes or even part of a minute. It was desirable and enjoyable because it kept sisters in touch with basic nursing care and let them use their practical skills and clinical expertise; it allowed them to do what they enjoyed — 'real nursing'. Teaching by example also provided opportunities to bridge the gap between school and ward, to relate practice and theory, and to assess standards of care and learner performance.

> We teach as we go along on the ward, we teach from the way we treat our patients. . . . I think this has a lasting impression. I teach when I work with them on the ward tidying up and making the patients comfortable . . . a better way than sitting giving them a good long lecture . . . that is what the school is there for.
>
> Sister White

The phrase 'teaching by example' was used generally for situations where sister and learners worked together giving direct bedside nursing care. It was suggested, however, that teaching by example could also occur when sister and learners were merely together in the same area with sister working alone, but visible and available to the learners. This form of teaching by example rested on the assumptions that learning would occur by osmosis and that the student would ask if unsure about anything. The main difficulty with this approach did not seem to be appreciated; that there are times when learners do not recognise their own learning needs and difficulties, and do not know the questions to ask. Sister White remarked: 'We always tell them that if they do not know anything, they have just to ask.'

Formal tutorials and lectures

Some sisters felt that it was possible to teach during or at the end of a ward report, during shift overlap periods in the afternoons, or at visiting times. On these occasions, teaching was often described as a 'formal tutorial' or a 'lecture'.

Ward report was felt to be a particularly good time to teach because it gave sisters the chance to provide reasons for nursing care and to assess students' knowledge and understanding of their work with each patient. Compared to teaching by example, lectures and tutorials were considered on the whole less enjoyable, more difficult to do, too time-consuming and less appropriate methods for sisters to use.

Sister Red remarked:

> I just can't get worked up about formal tutorials, that's what
> the school of nursing is for, but I do get worried about practi-
> cal demonstration and I'd far rather be on a late shift when you
> can get your sleeves stuck up and in with them to see what's
> happening. On the other hand, you want to be on an early
> shift for the administration, so you are torn.

Lack of time for teaching

Considering the very fragmented patterns of activity observed
(Appendix 2), it was easy to understand why the sisters felt that uninterrupted time for teaching was difficult to achieve within the
ward area. One sister remarked that it was 'virtually impossible' to
get peace to take a tutorial.

Even during ward report, considered one of the best situations
for learning, it could be difficult to fit the teaching in. For example,
in a ward of 30 patients, if only one minute per patient was taken
for giving information, and if time was added for discussion, questioning and 'teaching' related to the care of certain patients, plus
the inevitable time for interruptions, then 45–60 minutes could be
required for the whole session. Despite feeling under pressure during these sessions, and despite the frustrating interruptions, some
of the sisters did manage to teach and to create an environment for
learning during their reports.

Observation

It was mentioned in Chapter 3 that teaching, as a category of
observable behaviour, was difficult to define. Few teaching activities were recorded.

The teaching code was used when a sister gave a practical demonstration of care, or when explanatory information was given to
a learner following questioning and the discovery of gaps in knowledge. For example, while in the kitchen washing the cups one
evening, Sister Grey questioned a third year student about sar-
coidosis, provided information about a patient in the ward with that
disease and later questioned the student again in passing about the
information given earlier.

The teaching code was also used for tutorials and lectures. On a
Sunday afternoon during visiting, Sister Grey spent 36 minutes
uninterrupted in the treatment room out of sight of visitors, giving a
tutorial to two student nurses and an auxiliary. She spent the time
'going over the Kardex and case notes' and she questioned the learn-

ers about the patients' diseases and treatments; she was left in peace, because a staff nurse was available to talk with relatives.

Sister Gold spent 74 minutes out of her ward one afternoon, giving one of a series of tutorials to student nurses drawn from the wards of her own unit. Her subject was treatment and care of patients with anaemias. She disliked being away from her ward for so long on a busy day, but tolerated it because she had on duty a competent staff nurse who was to be in charge for the next two days while she had days off; Sister Gold felt that the staff nurse would get to know what was going on in the ward by being left in charge that afternoon.

Lack of knowledge, skills and confidence

The feelings about lack of time for teaching were closely linked to problems with what to teach and how to teach.

Formal tutorials and lectures seemed to consist of 'theory'. They dealt with diseases and their related anatomy, physiology, technical procedures and treatment, and the emphasis was mainly on medically orientated topics; the tutorials seldom focused primarily on nursing needs and care. It seemed that the sisters followed the pattern of teaching which they had experienced as students and they 'lectured' as they has been 'lectured to'. However, their remarks suggested that they realised that the subject material and the methods used were not altogether appropriate for ward-based teaching.

Some sisters said that the teaching of anatomy and physiology was not their job and should be done by the school of nursing. Sister Pink remarked:

I find it difficult to sit and tell them about a certain illness. . . . I do enjoy teaching the students by example when I am doing things with them.

It seemed that the sisters were most secure in their knowledge of basic nursing, which could be taught by demonstration, by 'doing' rather than by 'talking'; they were less secure about their knowledge of 'medical' and disease-related topics which had to be put into words and talked about.

Both these approaches had drawbacks. Important information about nursing topics might not be described and discussed when the emphasis was on demonstration and the medical topics were sometimes talked about in a vacuum without making clear their relevance to nursing care.

One sister remarked that studying for the Diploma in Nursing was her way of dealing with her lack of up-to-date knowledge, and it is interesting that the knowledge which she felt she needed was 'not about actual nursing care' but about anatomy, physiology and diseases of patients.

Muddle about the most appropriate knowledge base from which to teach and uncertainties about how best to use scarce teaching time were accompanied by lack of confidence in teaching ability. Several sisters felt ill-prepared for teaching.

> I find it very difficult to do. I think it's probably a certain lack of confidence in myself, because before I became a sister I had never been involved in very much teaching. It's just something you have to learn and force yourself to do. . . . I took a bit more upon myself as a senior staff nurse because I could see the need for it. But up to that stage I certainly hadn't, and I think it was partly lack of confidence and partly the feeling that I wasn't really very sure about what I was teaching. But you just have to get on and do it until it becomes easier.
>
> Sister Green

> The reason I don't teach them as much is probably because I lack confidence in myself as a teacher. I have always found this to be a great problem . . . it does bother me . . . I think it's improving the more experienced you become in dealing with the students.
>
> Sister Black

Lack of expert help

The sisters felt that they needed help to meet students' learning needs; all, except Sister Red, expressed dissatisfaction with their existing clinical teaching support.

There were several problems. It was felt that the clinical teachers did not visit the wards often enough and they did not 'belong' to wards or units. Some still joined the students from a particular block intake, wherever they were working in the hospital, and this system was disliked by the sisters as the clinical teachers were occasional 'visitors' rather than regular members of the ward team. It was felt that the clinical teacher should be allocated to a group of wards with a common specialist link, rather than to a group of students scattered throughout the hospital.

> In a busy ward it would certainly help if the clinical teachers came oftener . . . we very rarely see them.
>
> Sister Pink

We don't have area clinical teachers. We discussed this and they prefer just to have groups. It is improving — a few years ago we had a clinical teacher in the ward twice a year and that was it. This is very bad. The clinical teacher should be doing more. If they have done the course, then they are much more qualified to do the teaching.

Sister Black

Because the clinical teachers were based in the school of nursing, some sisters did not feel that they had any chance to coordinate or 'control' the visits of the clinical teachers to the wards.

Sister Blue felt that ward-based teaching should be a shared responsibility drawing together service, education and administration:

This is my hobby-horse. There are five people, according to Salmon, involved in teaching in the ward area: the school of nursing, the unit nursing officer of the service side, the clinical teacher, the ward sister and the staff nurse. Now, just tell me, who do we see? We don't see the school, we don't see the unit nursing officer, the clinical teacher comes once or twice in three to four weeks. Where are these other people?

Sister Blue also felt that instruction and immediate feedback about performance were particularly important, but difficult to provide because of lack of supervision by experienced trained staff; too often learners worked unsupervised:

Students are not getting pulled up at the time a thing happens ... if you catch them at it the message goes home much harder.

Sister Red found contact with learners and teaching less of a problem than her colleagues. Her lack of anxiety about her teaching role was related to having adequate clinical teaching support from a unit based clinical teacher, and to her longer experience as a sister. Over the years, she had got over her uncertainties and had found answers to her early questions about what to teach and how to teach. She considered the clinical teacher as a valued member of her ward team; as an expert with whom she could devise a planned programme of teaching based on identified ward teaching opportunities and student learning needs:

Teaching used to worry me a great deal, because there were no cut and dried rules and regulations as to what the sister had to teach them. It was left to the time and the enthusiasm that the sister had for teaching, whether she did any at all. At present it doesn't worry me as much as before, having the extra support. We have a clinical teacher and although all ward sisters must have contact and teach student nurses even if it is by example, I don't feel such a strain on me because I know there is one person appointed and employed to do that . . . you certainly know that at the end of an allocation all the nurses have had several days with the clinical teacher.

Sister Red's only anxiety concerned situations where pressure of work and lack of time prevented her from taking immediate action to guide or correct a nurse on-the-spot:

If the ward is very busy and you can see things that could be improved upon, and there doesn't seem to be time to stop and teach a nurse, it can be very worrying . . . You are so busy just getting through the next few minutes. . . . It's one thing teaching by example but there are some things you have got to draw the nurse aside for and formally teach her.

Sister Red seemed more in control of ward teaching through being able to coordinate the teaching input of the registered nurses in her team — staff nurses, sister and clinical teacher, all with different levels of expertise but able together to provide a range of specialist skills on a regular basis.

Sister Red was the most senior sister in the sample. She had a high level of educational attainment and several post-registration professional qualifications.

In contrast, the most junior and least experienced sister, Sister Pink, was much less clear about learner's needs and teaching opportunities and methods:

I don't really go in for teaching . . . I do give them lectures sometimes but I am not very keen on that way of teaching. . . . If you have got time you can go with the student nurses and show them how to do things properly . . . even then, it is up to them to improve their standards themselves.

Neither Sister Red nor Sister Pink was particularly worried about teaching and both gave low ratings and rankings to this problem statement. Their remarks suggest, however, that their reasons for not being worried about it and their ability to interpret the teaching role were quite different.

Difficulty assessing learners

Assessment of learners worried some sisters considerably but reasons for difficulty with this aspect of 'getting to know' the student were often oversimplified, being attributed to lack of time with learners and to being unable to 'work with' them. Underlying this problem were uncertainties about what to assess and how to assess.

Sister Gold said:

> I often don't have enough time. I often find when I come to write an assessment that I don't know the student nurse. I have to depend on the staff nurses to tell me what's going on. She may not have the standard I expect; if I had missed her first days, I may never know the girl.

Sister Blue tried to tackle the difficulties of assessment by analysing the learning opportunities in her ward and by structuring some of her contact with learners. She had set out the information and experience required by the students, and had identified assessment criteria in terms of ward environment, safety factors, emergency procedures, personnel, expectations, and the kind of nursing care commonly required by her patients:

> I like to be able to talk with them from time to time. I have a system whereby they have an orientation sheet; when they come to the ward there are things they're expected to know within the first four hours of the shift, for example the layout, fire equipment, emergency equipment, etc. There's a second section which they have to know within the first three days, for example who the ward team are, the physio, OT, chaplain, social worker, and they have a session with the ward sister or staff nurse about what is to be expected of them during the time and what experience they can gain. The third section they must find out for themselves, the management of valuables, accident forms, how to deal with visitors' complaints. I've got copies of the school of nursing report and they get one of those as near to half time as possible and I try to see them . . . but there's still a lot of room for improvement. I would like to discuss with the students how they feel about the ward, if they feel they are learning, and what they have learned; question them on why they are doing specific nursing care for specific conditions relating practice to theory.

Sister Blue's awareness of learners' needs and her more organised approach to contact with them did not result in low ratings for the statements about learners; rather, her perceptive approach seemed to make her more aware of the need for even better supervision of learners, and she gave the statements high worry ratings.

Sister Blue and Sister Red made two other important comments about relationships between sisters and their students. Sister Blue felt that it was important to give students a chance to say how they felt about their time in the ward. By encouraging a learner to analyse ward experience constructively, the sister could get feedback about her plan for each learner. Sister Blue therefore developed the concept of contact from being simply 'working with' the learner, to the idea of a planned, integrated programme for each student in the ward; a programme which would include, as one of its elements, 'working with' the student.

Teaching learners was also felt to be stimulating and a challenge because it made sisters think about and talk about their work. As Sister Red remarked, it kept her 'on her toes':

> At weekends I still like to work with student nurses. I certainly get an awful lot of stimulation from them and they keep you on your toes with the questions they ask . . . it's a two-way thing . . . I'm sure a sister would get very much more out of her job by teaching. There's no better way of learning your own subject and keeping up to date than by actually trying to express it to other people.

SISTER AS COORDINATOR

Interruptions

'Being interrupted so often', in tied rank position of 3.5 overall, produced high rankings and ratings for all but one sister, Sister Grey. Her solution to the interruption problem was unique. She kept moving, at speed:

> That could well be a problem particularly for junior sisters who don't have very much confidence. . . . There are certain interruptions you can't avoid but I keep them to a minimum. If I don't want to be interrupted I won't be.

Sister Grey felt that interruptions were 'not too much of a problem', not because they did not exist but because many could be controlled. She knew, however, that valuable contact with patients, relatives, nurses and others could be lost by controlling interruptions in a way which reduced her availability, and she realised that her way of working was not always in the best interests of good communication.

The sisters identified different types of interruptions. Overt or 'actual physical' interruptions were caused by people approaching sister or by the telephone. Covert interruptions were described neatly by Sister Red as 'occult interruptions in your own mind'. Interruptions could therefore be initiated by others and by sisters themselves as they responded to things observed, thought or remembered. The sisters did recognise that they often broke off whatever they were doing to attend to matters noticed in passing and it seemed that 'occult' interruptions were an inevitable part of the work of an alert, observant sister.

The fact that the word interruption had different shades of meaning underlined the difficulty of using observation as a method of recording the activities of sisters. The overt interruptions and activities could be seen and recorded. The occult interruptions could only be discovered through describing what it felt like to be doing the non-observable parts of a sister's work. Some sisters were able to describe the non-observable, and as they talked they identified an important skill possessed by experienced nurses. The skill was that of responding to patients, to the ward environment and to the activities of those in it with all the senses, selectively sifting and sorting sensory input both consciously and subconsciously. Accompanying this skill were problems of fragmented train of thought, of a mind full of facts and of half-remembered details; and from the fragmented thoughts in buzzing minds arose self-initiated activities which further fragmented a sister's work. The dilemma facing the sisters seemed to be that interrupting contacts and activities were often important and essential to ward communications.

The main difficulties with interruptions were their frequency and the fragmentation of thought and activity associated with them;

It is really there to some degree all the time, whether it's an actual physical interruption or whether it is this kind of occult interruption in your own mind . . . this constant feeling that you are never completing one thing that you've set about doing. Although you aren't actually interrupted, your mind is interrupted by thoughts, messages. A bell might ring, and although you might not have to go and answer that bell, it triggers off something. . . . Things that you see trigger off a reminder that such and such is to be done. . . . If you have too many interruptions very important things can get missed unintentionally. But you get to the stage where you simply cannot think without interruption and I've sometimes had to go away into the duty room and shut the door simply to think. It's the fact that it's so ongoing. It's with you all the time and that's the reason I've put it at the top.

Sister Red

It's just intolerable — we sit down for report; now, if you've got 34 patients and you spend two minutes only with each that equals 68 minutes; people knock at the door, visitors ask to see relatives, the domestic supervisor's complaining about the toilet, the auxiliary's complaining about something else, the ward clerkess constantly interrupts but she's got to answer the 'phone so she's got to interrupt. ... Sometimes I'm walking along the corridor and I don't quite know what I'm going for, I've forgotten what I was originally about to do because of interruptions.

Sister Blue

The sisters were often tired and sometimes exhausted using so much mental energy dealing with the 'occult' messages, in addition to using so much physical energy dealing with normal activities. Interruptions created a feeling of unfinished business, of doing too many things at the one time; a fear of forgetting things or of making errors, especially when the workload was heavy and staffing ratios poor. On such occasions, the combination of information overload and interruptions led to 'intolerable' situations in which sisters felt they were losing control.

Interruptions were also considered to be dangerous in certain circumstances. For example, during a drug round, a sister's attention would ideally be focused on checking the dosage and the distribution of correct drug to appropriate patient, especially when a student nurse was being instructed and supervised. However, interruptions upset concentration and one sister felt that to avoid accidents all ward and hospital personnel should be advised never to interrupt a sister during a drug round except in an emergency.

Observation

Observation revealed some of the problems associated with giving out medicines.

As the sisters moved from patient to patient with the drug trolley, many activities other than those directly related to drug administration intervened. Table 5.3 shows the number of drug-related and other activities recorded for each sister during an evening drug round. Most of the intervening activities were initiated not by

Table 5.3 Drug round activity pattern: number of drug-related and unrelated activities recorded for each sister during an evening drug round

Sister	Drug-related activities	Unrelated activities	Total	Time taken (min)
Gold	24	22	46	75
Green	17	14	31	24
Grey	28	19	47	38
Brown	15	14	29	27
White	19	12	31	14
Black	16	20	36	24
Pink	7	5	12	12

patients, nurses, doctors or others but by the sisters themselves. For example, the sisters attended to the comfort of patients, adjusting bedclothes and giving drinks; they checked charts and intravenous infusions; they observed patients and looked for nurses; they talked in passing to patients, relatives, doctors, domestics and porters; they wrote forms and made telephone calls.

During these drug rounds, it seemed that the sisters interrupted themselves more often than they were interrupted by others. Therefore advising others not to interrupt and distract a sister in the interests of safety would have been only a partial solution. Also, on the evenings observed, the patients, doctors, nurses and others would not have been able to consult a staff nurse first, as the sisters had only student nurses and auxiliaries on duty with them.

To change this fragmented pattern of activity at drug rounds and cut down interruptions, sisters would have to do more than advise others to approach another senior member of the nursing team, if available. They would have to alter their customary reaction of responding immediately to stimuli, instead storing the information for action after the drug round. However, this might be unrealistic and undesirable. A mind already full of detail might not be able to store readily new information gathered while going round the ward. On-the-spot action might reduce the chance of information overload; it might also be preferable in the interests of patient comfort and safety if, for example, a patient was uncomfortable, if an intravenous infusion was about to run through, or if a nurse required help or instruction.

The drug round example shows therefore that the interruption problem is complex and its solution more than a matter of stopping people talking to sister.

Availability

Remarks made about availability and about meeting the demands of many people were often related to the comments about interruptions. The statements 'Meeting the demands of so many people' and 'Being available to everyone while on duty' were ranked respectively sixth and seventh overall.

The dilemma of availability was clearly described. The sisters wanted to be available because it was through frequent contact and communication with the many people in their wards that they exercised their function as ward managers. Being available was stimulating and a necessary and inevitable part of the sister's coordinating role. Several sisters talked about the challenge of the 'linchpin' position. Dealing with all comers and struggling on with all the interruptions created a feeling of excitement. Being 'in demand' and the 'centre of attraction' was enjoyable. A sister could get a 'kick' out of coping, and the ability to meet demands provided job satisfaction and enhanced self-esteem.

> Meeting the demands of so many people can give you quite a satisfying feeling. . . . They respect you, they trust you and they take your word. They feel if sister tells them it means something.
>
> Sister Brown

> We tend to struggle on with the interruptions all around, but then I suppose that is what makes the job exciting . . . you are in demand, you are wanted. How much of it is meeting a need in ourselves? From a really selfish point of view, you are a centre of attraction. . . . It gives you a kick if you can send your customer away with the answer. So although it worries you a lot, it's an inevitable part of the job.
>
> Sister Red

> I like to feel that I am available to everyone, to the dietician, the patients, the doctors, the student nurses and everybody else, relatives as well. It's difficult because you are so busy you sometimes just haven't got the time. You like to be important to everybody. It's nice to feel you're the person everyone wants to see.
>
> Sister Green

Being identified as the 'key person' in the communication network, however, was difficult, and coping with the volume and varied demands of contact created pressure, conflict and frustration:

> It makes me feel frustrated, angry, useless, inadequate. So many people stop you in the corridor.
>
> Sister Blue

It gets extremely annoying. I suppose I have to be available otherwise I wouldn't know what was going on, but it can come to the extreme where every Tom, Dick and Harry insists on seeing sister and it may not be necessary.

Sister Gold

They all seem to want sister even although staff nurse is there. It's the frilly cap they want to see and that can be quite frustrating.

Sister Brown

It was difficult to provide the many different kinds of personal and professional 'support' needed by such a wide variety of people. Sister Red remarked:

It's just this feeling you are there to support everyone... the student nurse needs support, but so does the auxiliary who's got some home worry, so does the new staff nurse, so does the experienced staff nurse trying to stand up for herself. It involves so many other people, medical and paramedical staff, relatives, tradesmen, visitors, patients.... I think we don't often enough take people into duty rooms, shut the door and give them our undivided attention.

Some of the sisters suggested that there were priority groups of people to whom they should make themselves available; for example, patients and their relatives, and learners. However, being seen to be available and approachable when 'rushing around' was not easy, and when a sister was busy she could find that important contacts with patients felt like irritating interruptions. Sister Black remarked:

I try to make a point of seeing the patients at some stage of the day even if at times it's only to say hello, but I do find that difficult... they feel that the ward sister is always busy, always doing something. As one patient said to the consultant, 'Well, if I could get sister to stand still for five minutes.' I felt terrible — because I really had been rushing that morning and it was a wee simple kind of thing but obviously important to him. He had sat and worried about it... I remember thinking at the time, 'That's a trivial thing, two seconds of my time would have dealt with that.'

Exercising control over availability was difficult but, as Sister Blue suggested, it was not impossible. She felt that a sister's usual method of dealing with people, immediately, on the spot, was inefficient and created the unrealistic expectation that a sister would always be available to all comers. She suggested that in certain circumstances an appointment system should be used:

> There's no organisation. You fit round them, nobody fits round you. . . . I think we need to have more of an appointment system. You would never dream of expecting a patient to have an X-ray or physiotherapy without making an appointment. I had a drug rep. up the other day: 'Can I see you for a few minutes, Sister?' 'I'm very sorry. Not today, but I'd be happy to make an appointment.' He looked really indignant. I just think that the nursing service is totally taken for granted. You just cope with everything and we are just trying to do the impossible at times.

During the study, however, a situation arose in which an appointment system was unwittingly sabotaged by a conflict between expectations. Sister Brown was asked by her nursing officer at short notice to attend an afternoon meeting at a time when she already had appointments to see relatives and the liaison district nurse. She objected to this request but assumed that the meeting had to take precedence over her plans and she felt that the only problem was the one hour's notice. The nursing officer did not ask whether the time was suitable or whether sister had prior arrangements for the afternoon. The sister deferred to her senior's order; the nursing officer did not consult the sister about the use of her time, and the appointments were broken.

Another way of dealing with the problems of availability and the many demands of the job was to 'delegate' and to 'redirect' people to a staff nurse. Sister Green commented:

> It's difficult being available. You do get so many interruptions. There's a bit in that about training people to realise that sometimes you are not the person that they need to come to — maybe a staff nurse will do. So many people think the ward sister is the key person and everybody has to speak to sister if she's on. You'd want to be able to, but I'm sure there's a lot other people could do for you.

But this solution had its own difficulties. Several sisters realised that both the public and colleagues would prefer to speak to the sister. They would seek out 'the frilly cap' and might not be satisfied with a staff nurse's information. And the sisters themselves admitted that in certain circumstances the staff nurse might not have enough experience or knowledge to deal with matters adequately.

You can delegate more, but so often they just want to see sister. If you say that staff nurse is there and would you mind having a word with her as I'm busy at the moment, sometimes they are quite offended, and I suppose it takes more time redirecting them.

Sister Blue

Relatives don't think they've got the right information until they've seen the ward sister. A junior staff nurse may not understand what is happening, may not have the experience of handling relatives and may give the wrong side of the story or weight it the wrong way.

Sister Gold

It was also suggested that a ward clerk or receptionist could ease the demands on a sister. However, the comments about the usefulness of a clerk in dealing with the telephone and preventing interruptions reflected the optimism of the sisters who did not yet have a clerk and the realism of the sisters who had one.

It would be very nice to have a ward secretary who sat and dealt with all that.

The ward clerkess constantly interrupts but she's got to answer the 'phone so she's got to interrupt.

There were no simple or easy solutions to the problems of availability.

Too much to do

Several issues were raised by the statement 'Having too much to do every day', which was in tied rank position of 8.5 overall. For example, there was the question of expectations.

Sister Gold often felt that she had too much to do and she considered that others had unrealistic expectations about the amount of work with which a sister could cope:

Everybody expects you to do everything. In order to have good communications everybody comes to sister. I find it's just impossible to do everything, the administration plus the patients and student nurses. . . . The hours now are far too short.

She felt anxious, frustrated and under considerable pressure, yet it seemed to be hard for her to accept that her own self expectations might be very high, or that a review of work priorities might be necessary. All aspects of her work seemed important and she felt that she should be able to cope with everything.

Sister Red, the 'deviser of systems', did not feel as overwhelmed by work as Sister Gold. As a result she was able to comment more objectively, and suggested that the amount a sister did could be under her control as manager. In order to be seen to be in control and to feel in control, organisation and delegation were needed:

> It depends what you mean by too much. In any job you can go on finding more and more to do. It depends on what you set as your standard. In the present system of running most wards there would seem to be too much to do. Do we delegate enough? The more you can work at devising systems for any part of your work the more peace of mind you have as the manager. . . . If the people carrying out the job don't get through the work as quickly as you'd want, that's maybe not entirely your fault if at least you've devised a workable system. If you got terribly upset every day at how much you hadn't done, you would go off your head.

Sister White, who ranked this statement first and gave it maximum rating, had doubts about delegation. She felt that it was difficult and time-consuming to have to 'explain everything' to 'junior staff' and she felt uncomfortable when her work had to be done by less experienced nurses:

> You know that there are certain things you only can do and it is harder to leave someone else to do them, not so much if it is a staff nurse, but more if it is in an enrolled nurse. If the other sister is on, you know that you and she are tuned to the same wavelength. With somebody else, you have got to sit and explain everything that needs to be done.

Sister White's senior colleague disagreed, however, and felt that staff and enrolled nurses had to be given delegated work under supervision in order to learn. Sister Brown commented:

> It used to be that the consultants liked the senior sister always to be on the ward. We decided it was time this was stopping. It met with a wee bit of a long face at first; however, they got used to it and it works quite well. We let staff nurse do the main ward round but we find, to keep the atmosphere comfortable from the point of view of staff/consultant relationships, sister is usually there.

Sister White was worried for another reason about having too much to do. She mentioned on several occasions that her home life and her marriage took priority over work commitments and, when she was busy, there could be conflict between them. She felt under pressure knowing that she had to be off duty at 4 p.m. to catch the bus to be home in time to prepare her husband's meal before he left for evening work.

For Sister Blue the problem was fulfilling her teaching role when she had too much to do. Teaching was one of her priorities, but she felt that it should be a shared responsibility. She had tried to 'manage' the situation by seeking help from within her nursing team, from the nursing officer and from the school of nursing:

> If those tutors were in the ward they would be taking a lot off you. If the nursing officer was doing her bit she would be taking a lot off you. . . . So much of the teaching of students could be done by other people who *should* be doing it.

Sister Grey gave this statement lower rating because she enjoyed the challenge of coping with high workload. Her worry was not about quantity of work, but about poorer quality of work under pressure:

> If we are really short and really pushed — what bothers me then is not the fact that you have got so much to do and so few people to do it, but that you don't get the basic things done as you should. So it's not the amount of work, it's just that you tend not to keep up the same standard.

The idea that there was an optimum amount of work which sisters enjoyed and an optimum pace of work at which they would function well was raised once again by Sister Green when she talked about having too much to do:

> That only become a worry if I am really swamped with the work and get completely disorganised . . . It comes in fits and starts, busy spells and quiet spells. You prefer to be busy as long as it's not swamping.

Although the sisters often longed for quiet spells, they did not appear to have plans for using them and it seemed to be difficult to predict when they would occur. As a result they did not enjoy quiet times and felt that the time was 'wasted'. They either went off duty early to make up for all the extra time worked, or stayed and perhaps felt guilty because they were not busy. And it was Sister Pink, the least experienced sister, who noted the workload/staffing paradox:

> When you are really busy, all of a sudden all your staff disappear. The minute you go quiet all your staff appear again.

Fluctuating workload altered perception of adequacy of staffing even when numbers of staff did not change.

Peace and quiet

The statements 'Not having enough time to myself on duty' and 'Doing ward work in off-duty time' were given lower overall rankings of nineteenth and twenty-fourth respectively. Four sisters, however, did include these statements in their top ten problems, and their comments revealed not only why they needed peace and quiet, but also why it was so difficult to find it. Privacy and uninterrupted time seemed almost impossible to achieve within the ward area where activity and thought were so fragmented by interruptions of all kinds. Sister Blue remarked:

> It's not that I want to be away from people, I want to be with the students and patients and everyone as much as possible; but on the other hand you have got to have time to sit down and plan care and plan the day. . . . I often feel that half the trouble with the job is that I just do not have time to think.

The activities which required concentrated thought and attention included preparing student assessments and duty rotas, writing reports, talking in private to patients, relatives or staff, planning for change and working out teaching programmes.

Five sisters did not have an office of their own; they shared very small rooms with the medical staff, an unsatisfactory situation for the nurses and the doctors. But even when a sister had her own room, unless she locked the door or used a 'do not disturb' sign, certain activities could not be carried out there because of interruptions. Sister Black said:

> If I have to do reports I usually take them home because I have peace and quiet to do them. The duty room is like a thoroughfare — you are interrupted so many times.

The position of the sister's room within the ward area also influenced communication and interruptions, and one sister whose tiny office was situated next to the lift shaft had to cope with regular noise from lift operation.

It also seemed that there were few places available off the ward to which sisters could — or would — go to work. Off-the-ward activities, such as visiting a hospital library, seldom occurred.

Two sisters, however, did not see any reason to want or need time to themselves:

> On the whole, if I can get my day's work done in ample time that is all I want. I am not one to sit by myself.
>
> Sister White

I don't really think you are there to have time to yourself on the ward. You are there for the benefit of other people.

Sister Pink

Reactions to having to do work in off-duty time in hospital or at home varied from dislike to enjoyment. Sister Gold felt that ward work and shift work were demanding enough without having to cope with matters such as off-duty rotas in her personal time:

> It can be very annoying. . . . It may affect your social life and you've got unpredictable, unsocial hours as it is. If you don't get out of hospital life, you eat, sleep hospitals and ward work, therefore I think it's important that as far as possible you don't take ward work home.

In contrast, Sister Red preferred to do some of her work in off-duty time when free from the 'occult messages':

> There are quite a number of things I can do better in off-duty time. . . . On duty you haven't time and I feel I can't put my full mind to it.

Sister Grey was also quite happy to do ward work in off-duty time, but unlike Sister Red she did not take work home to get away from the bustle of the ward. Sister Grey extended the working day in the ward area by coming into the ward half to three-quarters of an hour before the shift started, particularly on ward round mornings, and she often stayed in the ward well after the end of a shift.

Sisters Brown and White did no work in off-duty time. They neither found it necessary nor wished to, therefore there was no problem. Sister Brown seemed to be able to fulfil the demands of the job, as she interpreted them, to her satisfaction within working hours and Sister White placed home commitments before work commitments. She said:

> That's no problem because I don't bring any work home. I don't believe in it. . . . I believe in getting off as soon as the clock strikes four. Somebody else is there to take over.

During observation, the number of times the sisters were observed working on their own was recorded. In a sense, this could be interpreted as time to oneself, but it was not possible to tell by observation how much of this time was spent on thinking and planning. It was found that as much as 23 to 39 per cent of total observed time was spent working alone but these times were made up largely of many short, frequently changing activities and brief, interrupted periods of time were not regarded by the sisters as suitable for thinking and planning.

It was clear that substantial periods of uninterrupted time were seldom available during a shift, and on the rare occasions they did occur, some of the sisters seemed to lack motivation, interest, ideas and energy to use the time constructively.

Sister Gold was one who did have clear ideas about how she would use extra time to herself. She said:

> I would build up teaching material . . . bring myself up to date, go to the nursing library — all of which is impossible.

However, when the quiet spells arrived, Sister Gold found that she often had neither energy nor inclination to get on with her plans and was only too glad to take time off.

It seemed that in order to find time on the job for time-consuming thinking and planning, several difficulties would have to be overcome. The sisters would have to alter their methods of work to create less fragmented patterns of activity — a difficult course of action; or they would have to secure periods of uninterrupted time by doing their thinking and planning out of the wards. But the sisters seldom left their wards. When they did, off-ward activities were usually considered as extras rather than as integral to ward management and patient care. Also, a sister would have to feel at ease when away from the ward. She would have to feel satisfied that there were competent staff available to provide adequate supervision in her absence; but even with adequate staff, some sisters seemed uncomfortable if unable to give personal supervision and see what was going on with their own eyes. It also seemed that some simply disliked being out of the ward at all, so accustomed had they become to being within its four walls.

It's not my job

The statement 'Doing things that are not part of my job' was ranked sixteenth overall.

Each sister gave an example of work she did which she considered was not part of her job, but reactions to doing such work were not always unfavourable and varied from annoyance and mild irritation to enjoyment.

Sister Grey spent time on non-nursing duties by choice. On early and late shift and even when domestic staff and junior nurses were available, Sister Grey was observed preparing tea for patients and washing up in the kitchen afterwards, doing rounds washing locker tops, renewing water jugs, emptying rubbish bags, and generally tidying up at bed areas.

Sister Grey knew that it would be difficult for an observer to record accurately non-nursing work. She pointed out clearly the impossibility of doing so by describing how apparently non-nursing activities such as washing lockers or giving out water jugs included important nursing activities — for example, while washing lockers she said she could observe, assess and talk to patients and be available to answer their questions; she could attend to comfort, adjusting pillows and bedding, and she could assess fluid balance and hydration.

Sister Grey need not have been involved in many of the domestic activities but it might have been difficult for her to break such a well-established pattern of working. Strict adherence to routine, meticulous attention to detail and willingness to work a considerable amount of extra time seemed to influence her pattern of work.

Activities recorded as 'non-nursing' for other sisters included washing cups at times when a domestic was present in the ward and arranging patients' flowers; however, not only did the sisters enjoy flower arranging but it was clear that they were skilled at it and that their skills were appreciated by the patients.

Sister Pink's views about the definition of non-nursing work were shared by several of her colleagues:

> It is very difficult to say what is not your job. Anything to do with the patient is your job. Everything you do is connected with the patient, even filling in books. I think you could reasonably employ other people for it but I don't think it is necessarily not your job.

Help with clerical work and ordering equipment and supplies would have been welcomed by some sisters. Sisters Gold and Black felt that it should be possible to assess average needs for certain supplies to free the sister from regular ordering and checking of stores and equipment. The sister's responsibility would then be to monitor supplies and to amend standard orders if needs changed:

> Ordering light bulbs and toilet rolls and things like that. I feel that it is a bit ridiculous having responsibility for the ill patients and yet having to order toilet rolls.

Several sisters felt that they became involved in 'non-nursing' work through trying to fill gaps in the services of other professionals to patients. Although irritating, filling gaps at the time seemed to be easier than finding time to discuss the problem with the group involved. Sister Gold often felt that she had to step in and take on doctors' responsibilities at the time of a patient's discharge to prevent delays and inconvenience to patient and relatives:

> It makes me frustrated. I do things for the doctors simply because I know that if I don't get them done, then the patient's going to suffer. He may be waiting to go home and I take it into my own hands to send down the Kardex for drugs because the patient can wait hours to get a doctor.

'Washing up' and 'clearing up' were also disliked, and Sister Red felt that the time had come to change the image of the nurse as 'clearer up' after others, especially doctors; clearing up should be a shared responsibility.

Sister Brown, who gave this statement a high rating and ranking, felt strongly that she should not have to cook patients' breakfasts each morning in the ward kitchen. She did the cooking because of the distance between the main hospital kitchen and the wards:

> If fried eggs are on the menu, they come up cooked but like rubber. It is nicer for the patients to have it cooked on the ward.

Sister Brown felt that a tray service for meals would be ideal:

> What I would like to see is a tray service in the wards . . . no setting up and no tidying away. Apart from telling the waitress where the patient is, you have nothing else to do unless you have patients to feed.

This comment highlighted a difficulty created by developments which were intended to simplify nursing duties and to remove from nurses supposedly non-nursing, time-consuming aspects of work. The introduction of plated meal and tray service can remove some waitress aspects of nurses' work at meal times, but it can also mean loss of important opportunities to use nursing skills in relation to each patient's nutritional needs. Such a service can easily lead to meal times becoming unsupervised occasions — occasions when an ill patient might receive an unappetisingly large portion, when the hemiplegic patient might get an unpeeled orange, or when an oedematous patient might be given a salt cellar. In the face of technology, nursing skills and knowledge need to be re-examined, restated and actively taught lest they become lost and undermined by 'progress'.

Sister Brown's colleague Sister White also gave this statement maximum worry rating and she ranked it as her second problem. Her difficulty was having to 'act up' for the nursing officer. She regarded this as an 'extra', outside her ward responsibilities; she disliked being out of her ward, and found it difficult to make decisions about deployment of staff within the unit. Reallocating staff was 'a strain', and moving nurses between wards to fill staffing gaps was unpopular. The annoyance she perceived among her colleagues when they had staff taken away raises questions, first about the criteria used by a sister and nursing officer to determine when a ward is 'quiet' or 'busy', and second about whether the sisters would have been able to use 'extra' staff constructively during 'quiet' times. Most of the sisters did not seem to have plans for quiet times, plans which might have justified the retention of their staff and which could have been set against the apparent priority of filling staffing gaps in other wards.

Friction between staff

This statement was ranked fifteenth overall. Friction seldom occurred, but when it did it caused considerable upset.

> Doesn't happen too often but when it does it can be very uncomfortable, especially if patients, or the successful running of the ward, are being affected.
>
> Sister Red

> It is a horrible thing to happen. It causes strain, and the patients do sense that there is friction.
>
> Sister White

Examples were given of situations in which friction had arisen between a sister and others — members of the nursing team, nursing officers, other senior nursing administration, school of nursing staff and doctors.

Sister–doctor friction was sometimes attributed to the personality idiosyncracies of doctors and was tolerated reluctantly. However, some of the episodes of sister–doctor friction were possibly due not so much to personality factors as to a sister's difficulty challenging a doctor's opinions or practices.

Friction between sister and her other nursing colleagues occurred when there were problems dealing with staff assessment, counselling and discipline. Within a sister's own nursing team, for example, unprofessional conduct caused great anxiety. When a member of staff in one ward repeatedly appeared on duty smelling of alcohol, the sisters felt that the action taken by the nursing officer and the senior nursing officer had been inadequate. They felt that they had been left with an unresolved problem and this caused friction between sisters and management. Sister White said:

> There is one member of staff that we would like to see off the ward. Unfortunately there is nothing we can do about it as the nursing officer says it is not fair to move her. We'd be getting rid of our worries to another ward. Perhaps the situation may resolve itself.

When dealing with the assessment of attitudes of nursing staff, registered or learner, some sisters felt that their evidence was not believed. Sister Black commented:

> I had a staff nurse who created a very bad atmosphere in the ward. I found it very difficult to deal with the problem. I actually had to go and see the principal nursing officer and bypass the 7 [nursing officer] and 8 [senior nursing officer] because I felt that I just wasn't getting anywhere.

Sister Pink felt that on occasions there had not been enough understanding, support or guidance from the school of nursing and the nursing officer when she and her senior sister colleague had considered a student nurse unsatisfactory:

> Obviously you want to give people a chance to begin with, to improve. But if they are not improving, they should be disciplined and eventually put out. I don't think industry would put up with that. I think management and the school need to put their foot down. . . . The whole point of assessment, to my mind, is that if they are not good enough then they do not qualify, but they don't seem to think this.

Friction was also thought to occur when morale dropped or when staff became tired. Increased workload or a high death rate lowered reserves of physical and emotional energy and affected standards of work, and in these situations a sister could become an interpreter of fluctuations in ward atmosphere and a mediator between her own nursing team and the senior nursing administration.

Sister Grey suggested that the answer to problems of friction between staff was to keep them busy:

> Not an outstanding problem. You do get a certain amount of friction but you can soon overcome that by keeping everybody occupied, keeping everybody busy.

It seemed that her own fast pace of activity was being used successfully as a coping mechanism to blunt awareness or prevent awareness of friction. Whether the fast pace of activity itself was acceptable, however, is debatable.

Tiredness

The sisters agreed that their work could be physically and emotionally tiring. Tiredness was described as an inevitable part of the job, but the extent to which it was regarded as a problem varied. The statement 'Feeling tired' was ranked twelfth overall and ranking positions varied from second to twenty-fifth.

Tiredness could be associated with a feeling of satisfaction. Sister Red remarked:

> It doesn't worry me that I feel tired on the ward. I think that's an inevitable part of nursing. There's a kind of satisfaction in feeling tired, as an indication that I've put something into it.

Both the married and the single sisters considered that they had a dual work role, with homes to run and families to look after in addition to their professional duties.

> It bothers me that I feel so tired . . . I think it's because the job is so demanding. Sometimes I just seem to feel permanently tired even on my days off. I feel I should be able to go home and cope with a house as well, which of course is ridiculous. . . . I certainly don't know how people with families do it.
>
> Sister Black

> Thinking about the work and running a home as well as doing a full-time job I am sure you get more tired. My husband helps quite a bit. . . . He shares in the housework, so in a way I am fortunate.
>
> Sister White

Early shifts following late shifts led to tiredness, especially when home was far from work or when transport was limited. On these occasions, some sisters had a shorter than average night's rest and did not feel refreshed in the morning.

> On a late shift you go to bed overactive and you don't sleep. You get up feeling tired. . . . You snap at people and you don't get a good working relationship.
>
> Sister Gold

The overactive mind at the end of a shift was also a problem. The process of thinking about past events, checking and sorting and sifting the day's information and happenings, could delay the unwinding at the end of the day.

> It's more mental tiredness at times than physical tiredness. After I have had a ward round and admitting day, it takes me some while to unwind; my mind is still on the ward. . . . You tend to think for a long while after you have come home, 'Have I told them everything?'
>
> Sister White

The sisters talked of spacing days off and holidays, to avoid long periods without a break.

> If I have a long stretch between my holidays, I feel myself getting tired and 'crabbit'. You tend to lose your patience . . . you feel yourself being a bit more intolerant of people.
>
> Sister Pink

> Before I went on holiday, I was tired and I suppose inevitably it affects whatever you are doing in the ward. You tend to opt out a bit and get frustrated more easily.
>
> Sister Green

General health problems also caused tiredness and anxiety. Sister Gold knew that her health did influence her ability to cope, and she felt that this was not always understood by her senior colleagues. When a build-up of tiredness occurred, it could become difficult to distinguish between 'good' and 'bad' days; every day could seem 'bad' when tired and struggling to cope:

> A ward sister is not human almost. She's got to go on irrespective; she can't break down; she can't be tired. People don't stop to think that there might be sheer tiredness or worry on your own part and that you might have your own problems. I think that is a big factor in how competent and how efficient you are.

In her busy, medical ward with its inconvenient layout, Sister Blue found that dealing with administrative work alone was tiring. When in addition she had to help with clinical work, coping with combined responsibilities became exhausting. She said:

> I get absolutely shattered. I get sometimes to the end of the day and I can't think straight and I would really probably be better off duty. If you were just administrating or just doing the physical work, but you are doing both. . . . At my interview, Miss X said, 'Aim never to get into a situation where the

practical work is dependent on you.' That happens every evening shift: you are part of the basic workforce and running the ward at the same time.

The sisters' comments revealed, therefore, that tiredness was important, not only from the point of view of a sister's health and welfare as an employee, but also in relation to her ability to function competently and safely at work.

It was suggested that tiredness could be related to several factors: the number of patients in a ward and the amount of information about them to be assimilated; the number of staff to be supervised and supported; fluctuations in workload and staffing; the size of a ward and its layout; the kind of nursing care provided, and the level of stress inherent in it — for example, intensive care and terminal care; the self-expectations of the sister regarding her performance and her ability to cope; the sister's general health; other work and home and family commitments.

SISTER AND THE NURSING OFFICER

Rankings and ratings for the statement 'Getting the nursing officer to understand the ward' varied widely. It was ranked eleventh overall.

It seemed that the sisters liked and accepted a nursing officer who 'knew' the ward, who provided 'information', who 'understood difficulties' and who was 'available' when problems arose.

These positive attributes were mentioned only in vague terms. The appreciation of knowledge, the supply of information, the understanding of difficulties and the dealings with problems were not described in detail; and at the negative end, acceptance of the nursing officer was based on non-interference in ward matters. Sister White remarked:

> It really isn't a problem. We have a very good nursing officer. He doesn't interfere with the running of the ward.

From the criticisms of other sisters, it is possible to see the ways in which they felt a nursing officer should contribute to a ward. The nursing officer was not seen to be available as a clinical adviser or specialist. She seemed to have lost credibility, being described as 'out of touch', and as a result she was not regarded as someone who could offer support or understanding when the sister was under stress:

> . . . a big problem. They are just not on the ward enough. Even

although they offer to make a few beds, they can't understand the pressures — that you may have things building up and everything may happen at once. Also, they may have been out of the ward situation for a long time and things may have changed incredibly in the past two years.

                                                                Sister Gold

They forget what it is like to be in the ward situation. They forget the stresses and the coping.

                                                                Sister Blue

Failure to 'understand' the ward and its pressures was attributed to lack of time in a ward, to lack of involvement in clinical work or to being in a rush, which inhibited discussion and exchange of ideas. Sister Gold said:

> I feel I am frustrated. At present she rushes in and rushes out with an aura of hurry and there is no leisure about it.

Several sisters worried about fluctuations in staffing and workload. They felt that when the nursing officer looked at this problem 'numbers' of staff and patients were seen to be important, while 'quality' in terms of grade and competence of staff and dependency levels of patients was not taken into consideration:

> At times I feel that they don't fully appreciate the workload, having left the ward situation. You can have a full ward of 20 patients and not be as busy as a ward with ten. Sometimes I feel they come in and ask you a number and that's it. They don't seem to take into account how heavy you are.

                                                                Sister Blue

Sister Blue also felt strongly that clinical and teaching components of the nursing officer role had not been developed. She would have liked to discuss clinical problems with the nursing officer, using her as a clinical specialist in the nursing officer's own area of expertise and as a clinical adviser in general:

> The nursing officer's job is not practised as it was ever meant to be. There is no clinical participation whatever. . . . She is corridor orientated. I have had pressure area problems and was just flummoxed to know what to do. I would have liked to use her as a clinical expert.

Some sisters talked about being vaguely aware of the fact that changes had occurred in their wards which affected the nature and pace of their work. The nursing officer was not seen as someone who could help to interpret change, or offer support in the face of it, or make predictions and plan for future change. Sister Blue had noticed that the nursing officer could understand and help with a sudden acute problem, but she could not identify the nature of slow, steady trend of change. As a result, in the face of the nursing officer's apparent lack of understanding that change was occurring, she felt that she was just 'nagging' about problems, and eventually felt a sense of failure and loss of control:

> When there is an acute problem she can see it for herself. What is difficult is to get her to understand ongoing problems — a slow trend — if the work is just getting harder over a period. Then you just seem to be constantly nagging and nagging and it seems to have no effect. And then you start thinking, 'I'm failing, I'm losing control.' I would like her to note trends independently and perhaps tell *me*.

Closely related to these remarks about the nursing officer were comments from the statement 'Finding someone to turn to when I need help', ranked twentieth overall. Sister Pink, the most junior sister, looked to her senior sister for help. All the other sisters identified the nursing officer as a possible source of help, but they noted that her availability alone was not enough.

> You can always get hold of the nursing officer; they certainly are accessible, but action isn't always forthcoming.
>
> Sister Blue

The sisters indicated that they would have liked help from a nursing officer in these aspects of their work: personal counselling about their performance; support in the long term and in short-term crisis and stress; redeployment of staff when workload and staff numbers fluctuated; participation in clinical work; specialist advice on clinical matters; teaching learners; staff counselling and assessment; identification of changing trends; and analysis of problems.

Sister Red's approach to getting help was rather different from that of her colleagues. She seemed to be a problem solver and she talked with enthusiasm about trying to analyse work difficulties by herself. She felt that there could be alternative solutions to problems and she tried to work out who would best be able to help. She regarded the nursing officer as 'a sounding board' with whom problems could be shared and discussed, rather than as a person to whom problems would be handed over for solution:

There's always someone to turn to, nursing officers having been allocated to a unit with a bleep . . . often what you need is just someone to share it with, a sounding board. This is part of the job I really like: trying to decide who you get; sitting down with the problem; breaking down the problem, saying, 'Which book would I look up?' or 'Who knows the answer to this?', 'Who's had experience of this?' in the ward or the hospital or outside; or, if I were presented with the problem in the community, 'Who could I contact?'

Only one sister, Sister Brown, identified strongly enough with the nursing officer role to consider applying for promotion to that grade. It is interesting, however, that she seemed to feel happier than her colleagues about her own role as ward sister. She had a large number of low-rated problem statements and she tended to make fewer critical remarks about her own job at the time of the study.

SISTER AND THE DOCTORS

Of the two statements about doctors, 'Disagreeing with a doctor's instructions for a patient' caused the greater concern. 'Getting the doctors to listen to my point of view' was ranked twenty-second overall, but disagreeing with instructions was in the higher tied rank position of 13.5.

Conflict — care versus cure

Great strength of feeling and real distress were conveyed by some sisters as they talked about their disagreements with medical opinion and medical treatment. The main areas of conflict concerned the care of the terminally ill, the management of pain and relief of symptoms, and the care and resuscitation of elderly patients.

This does not come up all that often but when it does you can feel very, very unhappy about it. . . . When patients are to be given further treatment, subjected to tests that may cause them physical or mental pain, particularly when the nurse cant't really see the point of it. In elderly people, or people who are perfectly obviously dying, you begin to wonder if it is just an academic pursuit. I think that's when it upsets a sister most of all. If all the doctors are in total agreement with whatever the line of action is and you are the only person apparently disagreeing, it takes a brave ward sister to stand up and say, 'Give me ten good reasons why you want to do that?'

Sister Red

Younger doctors are very diet conscious. They see an obese old lady — it doesn't matter that she is 88 or 90 — and put her on a diet. I feel, and the head dietician agrees with me, that if Granny has lived to 88 or 90 and enjoyed her porridge and her pudding and her fish and chips, then leave Granny alone.

Sister Brown

These comments indicate not only the conflict between the value systems of nurses and doctors, but also the difficulties of speaking out and expressing doubt about treatment to medical colleagues, who are seen to be more powerful than nurses in the professional hierarchy.

The nature of the relationship between the sister and a doctor could be influenced by the doctor's level of seniority. Some sisters felt that they had the power to advise and, to some extent, control the work of junior doctors; with senior medical colleagues, however, a sister might have to prove her worth over time and be 'accepted' before her views would be respected. Even then, it was felt that a nursing viewpoint did not necessarily carry much weight against medical opinion. Sister Red remarked:

You just have to wait until you are established in your ward, accepted; until the point is reached where the doctors realise that you have valid points of view.

The nursing viewpoint
Sister Blue seemed to be the only sister who felt able to exchange views freely with medical staff. In her discussions with doctors, she tried to interpret for them the nurse's contribution to care and the distinction between nursing and medical viewpoints. For example, she was convinced of the value of the skilled observation of the experienced nurse in patient assessment, but she felt that the worth of such nursing skill was not well understood or acknowledged by some medical colleagues:

You've got to get across to them the importance of nursing. They'll quote biochemistry and haematology to you, and it makes no difference if the patient is cyanosed and looking unwell and got that grey look. How do you get this across to them? What is it a nurse can see in a patient which isn't necessarily displayed by his pulse, blood pressure or respirations? I've tried this several times but they've said that the potassium is okay and his sodium is back to normal, so he must be on the mend; and yet there's something niggling and quite often you are proved right.

Other sisters who thought that they could express their points of view freely and who did not consider this a problem seldom seemed in fact to exchange views with doctors or to debate areas of conflict. They also did not seem to have a clear picture of the nurse's contribution to patient care, as this remark by Sister Pink shows:

Our work is based on how our surgeons want their patients nursed.

Getting doctors to listen to a sister's point of view was therefore rated less of a problem for several reasons: firstly, because areas of conflict were being discussed and dealt with successfully; secondly, because sisters did not realise the nature of the problem or feel that there was conflict; and thirdly, because sisters were resigned to the inevitability of the difficulties after repeated attempts at tackling them had failed. Sister Grey talked of feeling frustrated, powerless and disillusioned as a result of longstanding disagreements and unsuccessful attempts at discussing problems with medical colleagues, and she had become resigned to living with differences of opinion.

LEARNING THE JOB

Three statements showed the difficulties of the traditional way of learning about the sister's job through on-the-job experience and off-the-job management courses. 'Considering myself as manager' and 'Getting the staff nurses to understand the sister's role' were ranked together in tied position of 17.5 overall, and 'Understanding my job responsibilities' was ranked in last place, twenty-fifth overall.

Although ranked last and generally less of a worry, understanding the job was a considerable problem for some sisters. They knew clearly what they were doing in terms of the daily routine and tasks to be completed, and in that sense they were familiar with the job and 'understood' it. However, at interview most of the sisters had great difficulty talking about their role as manager; they seemed vague about the nature of the job and its responsibilities and found it hard to describe.

Sister as manager
One sister found it difficult to regard herself as a manager in any
way.

> You do not think of the ward sister being a manager because I
> suppose you think of a manager as somebody who runs a de-
> partment store.
>
> Sister White

Some of the other sisters seemed to accept the word manager because it was such a commonly used term rather than because management was seen as integral to patient care. Dealing with ward
administration as 'manager' and being involved in clinical work as
'nurse' could be regarded as unrelated aspects of the sister's role.

> Some days I feel I am more a manager than a nurse.
>
> Sister Black

> I don't really consider myself as a manager. I am not very in-
> terested in administration. I do prefer the practical side.
>
> Sister Pink

Three sisters were able to see a relationship between management
concepts and their work as clinicians and as leaders of the nursing
team. These three, Sisters Red, Gold and Blue, were the most highly qualified academically and professionally. They had found their
management training relevant and helpful, and they were actively
involved in continuing education. They felt that it was not only 'the
ward' that had to be managed, but patient care itself. And in her
remark, Sister Blue brought together the concepts of the manager
and the nurse:

> A nurse is a manager from the moment she enters training but
> it's unconscious at first, it's not formal. When you plan a bed
> bath or a procedure, you manage it . . . I think that's how man-
> agement starts in nursing.

Off-the-job courses
Each sister had attended a three- or four-week first line management course and two sisters had also been to a six-week middle
management course. Despite their management training, some sisters, especially the junior ones, had great difficulty seeing management concepts as relevant or useful.

Management courses were described as 'a waste of time'. They
were enjoyed as a break in routine and as an opportunity to dis-

cover that others experienced the same problems. Course content was 'interesting' but 'abstract' and hard to relate to the reality of ward life. Sister White remarked that she 'just did not see any point in it'. Sister Grey had attended first line and middle line management courses and found them helpful; however, during observation it became apparent that she interpreted management by objectives to mean time targets — for example, taking 30 minutes to make all the beds before the consultants' round:

> The thing about management by objectives — that was what I found most helpful, because I do try and set myself a target and times to do it in. I don't always get there, as you know.

This interpretation of a school of management had thought-provoking consequences in practice (p. 40).

On-the-job experience

Each sister talked of having learned about some aspects of the sister's job, when they were students and staff nurses, through observing sisters at work. Watching and listening to the role model and being 'left to get on with it' were seen as the main ways of learning the role. Sister Blue said:

> The sooner you leave them in charge to get on with it themselves, the better. The answer is to get them to take the responsibility pretty smartly and they soon learn.

It was felt that length of time in the post was the most useful factor in learning the job and that understanding of the sister's role would grow with experience. When talking about the responsibilities of the job, Sister Green remarked:

> It's funny — you hardly think about them. It's not that you are not aware of them, you just come to accept them. As you get more experienced, it's just something that you come to know.

Job descriptions were of little help. Sister Gold said:

> You get a job description but it doesn't describe what a ward sister does. You've got to learn by hit and miss.

Learning by 'hit and miss' had its problems, however, as Sister Red so clearly described. Her words 'blunder', 'mistakes', 'distress' and 'bitter experience' indicated that the cost to a sister and to patients could be high:

As you blunder through things, make mistakes, get a red face, see distress — for example, amongst relatives who weren't summoned early enough: from every situation you learn. As a first-year ward sister it was difficult knowing what authority I had, knowing exactly my place, knowing what I could expect of other people, knowing what say I had in matters, how much I could take a stance beside the medical staff. I found it difficult to know how much I had to push myself forward to make a contribution.... I've come through the bitter experience of, for example, not calling relatives early enough or not speaking up early enough on a ward round about some nursing point.

It was felt that a staff nurse might be aware of the status, or 'place', of the sister, but she would not necessarily understand the duties and responsibilities of the role, or how to deal with them, unless she was actively taught. 'Leadership', 'delegation', and 'team communications' were regarded as difficult areas to understand and teach.

Several sisters recalled how difficult it had been for them, when staff nurses, to understand 'what all the trained staff used to do in the office all day long'. Simply watching the sister had not been enough to allow them to understand decision-making, and the mysteries of administrative aspects of ward management and patient care.

I couldn't understand why sisters spent so much time in the duty room. It's not until you actually become a sister that you realise the full responsibility.

Sister Black

During observation it was found that the sisters did spend considerable amounts of time in their offices, the range being from 34 to 45 per cent of their total time.

The most junior sister remarked that she had seldom discussed her work with the staff nurses because rapid turnover made it impossible; staff nurses 'stayed only a month or two' and therefore there wasn't 'much chance of teaching them anything about ward sisters'.

It could have been, however, that the difficulty was not so much having too little time to teach but uncertainty about what to teach and how to teach staff nurses about the sister's work.

Relying only on learning by experience and by observing a role model might well be a slow process, and the sisters' remarks did suggest that there was an urgent need for short-term, effective teaching on-the-job of the essentials of ward administration and clinical management.

KEEPING UP TO DATE

Continuing education

'Keeping up to date with new trends' was in tied rank position of 13.5 overall. Some of the remarks prompted by this statement are disturbing and they reinforce the current concern in nursing about continuing education for all registered nurses and for ward sisters in particular.

The comments show how the phrase 'new trends' was interpreted and the ways in which the sisters kept up to date. They also reveal their views about the gaps in their knowledge.

The sisters seemed to worry most about new trends and changes in medical treatment, in surgical techniques, and in drug therapy; several sisters also felt that their knowledge of anatomy and physiology was inadequate.

> Nowadays things have become so technical. There are so many new drugs, so many new techniques and the doctors sometimes fail to realise that you do not know that something is new.
>
> Sister Gold

Some sisters did not seem to appreciate that there might also be changes in nursing knowledge and practice, and on the whole there appeared to be less anxiety about keeping up to date with new trends in nursing itself. Sister Brown remarked: 'Basic nursing care has not changed and I don't think it will change.'

Knowing about new trends in nursing seemed to depend largely on the sister's level of interest and motivation towards seeking information actively herself from books, journals and colleagues. In contrast, knowing about changes in medicine, surgery, drugs and technology seemed inevitable and could hardly be avoided because these changes impinged directly on the sister's day-to-day work with patients.

Sister White gave this statement a higher rating than her colleagues, and she clearly had several worries:

> I would like to keep up to date but I do not know how. They have study days for sisters but I think they are a waste of time.

I think most of the sisters agree with this — they discuss nothing. In fact, I can't remember what the last study day was.

When asked if she could recall anything relevant from study days, she said:

We did have a man from insurance who frightened the life out of us. I suppose he did show us how people can sue. We should be open to ideas, but I suppose the only way is by learning from your wards. The doctors bring you up to date with drugs. Sometimes it does worry me that I do not know very much about new methods. The only way, I suppose, is by getting nursing magazines but I don't think I will learn very much from them. I did buy for a while, but I suppose I grudged the money: half of it was adverts and in the other half there were a lot of things that did not apply.

In contrast, Sister Green's remarks showed that she was strongly motivated towards keeping herself up to date. She seemed to be aware of changes in both nursing and medical practice and of their interdependence, and she felt that there were several sources of information available:

. . . Getting magazines, making use of study days, listening to the doctors and just being interested in what they are doing. We are fortunate here because there are a lot of meetings we can go to. I think if you are interested in continuing education then you will be interested in keeping up to date.

Each sister bought, or had access to, a nursing journal; although available, the journal might not be read.

I don't say I always manage to get round to reading it.

Sister Black

I don't really go in for a lot of reading. At home I want a change from nursing.

Sister Pink

The four sisters in the pilot study hospital seemed to be more actively involved in keeping up to date. Sister Green actually used the term 'continuing education' in her remarks; Sister Red had completed the Diploma in Nursing, and Sister Blue and Sister Gold were studying for the second part of the Diploma. The three Diploma sisters had higher levels of academic attainment in terms of numbers and grades of certificates held.

Being more aware of the need to keep up to date seemed to increase rather than lessen anxiety about it. For example, Sister Red remarked:

> Quite a worrying thing . . . there's keeping yourself from getting rusty and keeping up to date with *new* trends. So much of the time you spend encouraging other staff to go away and learn things, and are the very last to go yourself.

The need to promote the image of the sister as a knowledgeable person was both a problem and a motivating factor in keeping up to date; the self-image and the image in the eyes of nursing and other colleagues had to be maintained. Sister Gold said, 'It doesn't look good at a report if sister doesn't know.' It could be hard to admit gaps in knowledge, and Sister Red remarked that she preferred to be 'one step ahead':

> If something new is introduced, you ask questions about it and you try and master it yourself before letting the rest of your staff get it.

Sister Blue felt that sisters were sometimes unrealistic in their expectations about the breadth of their knowledge. She felt that specialisation was needed and that nursing expertise could and should be developed and shared within a hospital. She had often been aware of gaps in her own knowledge and skills, and she had wanted to seek help from nursing consultants when problems arose:

> If you were a doctor, you would call in the consultant specialising; a vascular surgeon would never dream of treating his own diabetic patients. So why is it that nurses feel they must be up to date with everything? I think we feel guilty because we don't know . . . nurses should specialise and seek advice. I feel that if I had a surgical problem in a medical ward, perhaps I could ring the sister or the nursing officer for the surgical area. I've been in desperation to know how to treat someone's pressure sores. Eventually I discovered the current treatment on the surgical side, by accident, at the lunch table.

Introducing change

Although the statement 'Making changes in the ward' was given low ratings and ranked twenty-first overall, the sisters were able to describe several difficulties associated with planning and implementing change.

The sisters differed in their ability to see the need for critical review of nursing practice. Some sisters were trying to introduce new ideas, the most frequently mentioned area in which change had been attempted being 'ward routine'. Others either did not regard this as an important part of their work or had become resigned to the fact that change was fraught with too many difficulties. Sister White remarked:

> I don't have a problem. We have been lucky, we don't need to make much change in the ward.

Change could upset routine, threaten a sister's popularity and create feelings of insecurity.

> You can't go into a ward and say, 'I am going to change this, and this. . . .' People won't accept it. You are going to be very unpopular.
>
> Sister White

Planning and implementing change could be very time-consuming and might be of low priority when a sister was busy getting through the demands and pressures of each day's work.

> As long as you've got a routine that's working, as long as the work is getting done you tend perhaps not to stop and think: 'Can I improve? Things have changed and therefore perhaps I should be making changes.' If the pressures get too hard, you deal with the immediate priorities.
>
> Sister Gold

Change could also be a very slow process. A single project might take years to complete, and waiting for the rare 'quiet times' or 'spare moments' to plan and to introduce new ideas was unrealistic, as these times were 'abnormal' and seldom used effectively.

Several sisters mentioned the difficulty of 'eradicating tradition'. The bigger the nursing team, the more difficult it became to discuss the new ideas with everyone involved and to get the changes implemented by the whole team.

> One of the hardest things I've found is eradicating tradition. In fact, thinking up the new system isn't nearly as hard as actually stopping people doing a procedure that they've done at 6 a.m. for the last 25 years.
>
> Sister Red

I met difficulty when I was new — certain members of staff had been in with the bricks. When I came at first — after every meal, stacks of bedpans were trundled into the wards on a wooden trolley. The bedpans were used and urine was measured there in the middle of the ward. I thought it must be very embarrassing for the patients. Now the patients get their bedpans when they need them and there is no bedpan trolley. The student and pupil nurses were very good; they adapted; but the older members of staff — I found out that when I was not there, this wooden trolley was being trundled into the ward just the same, so I put it out.

Sister Brown

One sister was cautious about introducing change. Sister Blue had been trying to move from task-oriented to patient-centred care, but she felt that the process and the outcome of change had to be carefully evaluated as there might be advantages in some of the 'old-fashioned' methods:

When I started, I just left things for about two months to see how it went. There were certain things I wanted to change: I wasn't very keen on mouth care rounds as such. I prefer them to do it as part of total patient care. On the other hand, there's a lot to be said for a mouth care round as they darn well go round and they do it. There's a lot to be said for some of these old-fashioned methods.

The perceived authority and control of senior nursing management could also influence the sister's position as change agent. A sister might not 'feel free' to introduce change, and change could be 'imposed'.

A new intensive care unit was to be developed in one ward, and the two sisters had been asked for their opinions about it at an early stage in the planning. They had wanted to take an active part in decision-making about the unit, but they felt that they had no real say in the matter, not only because they lacked information as a basis for discussion, but also because they were 'low' in the administrative hierarchy. As a result, senior nursing management were felt to be imposing unwanted change:

I put forward ideas . . . they asked for our opinions. The only people who were not keen were the ward sisters, but we were told we were having it.

Sister Black

Isolation

The statement 'Feeling isolated from other ward sisters' was ranked twenty-third overall. Two types of isolation were identified: geographical isolation within a ward area or unit, and professional isolation from peers and other nursing colleagues.

Sister Red, the most senior sister and the one who rated this statement highest, raised important points about peer contact. She felt that contact was needed, not just for moral support, but also for exchange of professional knowledge and skill:

> I feel quite strongly about this. On many wards there is only one ward sister and she can feel very alone in her job. We can gain an awful lot from sharing, in keeping up to date with procedures, trends in nursing, what's going on in the training of students, and so on. I think you can get an awful lot of moral support from your own sister colleagues . . . you can't share that with your staff nurse, with your doctors, with your patients or with your family, because they don't understand. If there is no formal contact with your colleagues, it gets done in a very hurried way over meals or giving a person a lift home. It comes very low on the list of priorities, and I think that's a big mistake . . . there's an awful lot to be gained from sisters in other specialities and subjects. We should use each other.

Sister Gold described the job as 'very lonely':

> The staff nurses can turn to each other or to the ward sister and ask for help; the student nurses can turn to the trained staff for help and guidance; but it's not easy for a ward sister to turn to the nursing officer and discuss things.

Sister Gold's final comment about her feelings of failure was disturbing:

> One or two times I've felt I was failing, and there was no one I could really go and talk it over with. You can't discuss work outside the hospital either, therefore you can't get rid of a lot of the pressures and worries. Sisters now mostly live out — perhaps living-in had that advantage.

Sisters' meetings did give opportunities for getting together with colleagues, but they seemed at times to be little more than grievance sessions and they did not provide much practical help with problems. However, as Sister Black remarked, the airing of grievances did at least provide a common bond between sisters:

> There is very little contact between the wards. We go to sisters' meetings but that is all. It's nice to know that you are not

running a one-man battle, that all the other ward sisters are facing the same problems.

Two sisters did not feel isolated. Sister Green worked closely with the sister in the adjoining ward and had opportunities to talk over problems. There seemed to be less social and professional isolation in this unit owing to its compact geographical layout. Sister Brown did not feel isolated as she enjoyed the informal, social aspects of contact with other sisters in her unit while 'doing the block', standing in for the nursing officer:

> I do not feel isolated at all. . . . If you are on the block and you go round the sisters, they all have time to speak to you and you can talk about various things — it does not necessarily have to be about the hospital. I find the atmosphere really great.

The junior sister in that same ward, Sister White, felt quite differently about contact with the other unit sisters. She talked of contact as 'chat' and 'gossip'; she preferred to stay in her own ward, and she was content to be isolated at work because her home life provided all the social contact she needed.

Two other sisters were happy in their isolation.

> I suppose in some ways we are isolated. We tend to go our own way on the ward, but I don't think that's of any importance.
>
> Sister Grey

> Does not really bother me. I never see any of them. I live in my own wee world.
>
> Sister Pink

6

Summary and conclusions

The nine sisters in this study provided a wealth of detail about their day-to-day work which richly illustrates its complexity and its difficulties.

It would be unwise to generalise about the problems of sisters as a whole on the basis of such a small sample. Nevertheless, the in-depth case-study approach with only a few individuals proved to be valuable for several reasons. It revealed a number of ways in which the competence and welfare of sisters can be adversely affected by their problems at work. It also highlighted some of the potentially important differences which exist between nurses who occupy the sister grade. For example, the nine differed in professional and educational background, in their understanding of their role responsibilities, in their perception of and response to work difficulties, and in the context of their social and family commitments into which the work role had to fit.

In one thought-provoking respect, the two parts of the study differed. On-the-job, comparatively few problems were identified and discussed and most of the sisters' comments were about 'getting the day's work done'. At the end of a shift, the sisters seemed preoccupied, as though mentally working through a checklist of finished and unfinished business. As a result, when they were interviewed on-the-job, some of the sisters found it difficult to give their full attention to considering the ups and downs of the day.

However, when the sisters were interviewed off-the-job, away from the ward area and when free from immediate work demands, a wider range and greater depth of comment was obtained and it became apparent that at the time of the study the sisters were experiencing many other problems which had not been mentioned on the job.

The striking difference between the two occasions suggests that giving careful consideration to time, place and preoccupation level could influence the success of a discussion between, for example, a sister and her nursing officer. Freedom from distraction and freedom from worry about 'What's going on?', 'Who's in charge?' and

'How are they all coping?' might increase the likelihood of getting to grips with important issues and problems.

Fragmented activity — the way sisters work

In this study, the considerable fragmentation of nurses' work was confirmed. Approximately three-quarters of the sisters' activities lasted for less than 2 minutes and approximately half lasted less than 1 minute (Appendix 2).

Why is the work of nurses so fragmented? Is their pattern of behaviour learned simply from watching and imitating other nurses? Are nurses so forgetful or such poor planners that they fail to think through activities clearly from start to finish? Is it because other people interrupt so often? Or is their disjointed way of working, which can be so mysterious to a non-nurse observer, related in some way to an acute awareness of the working environment?

Analysis of the interviews and the observations revealed several factors which influenced the sisters' patterns of work, factors such as availability, interruptions, the ability to remain in control, and the level of the sister's sensory awareness.

Availability, interruptions and control

Being available was regarded as a professional necessity and it was enjoyable. The sisters wanted to be available because they recognised that getting the information needed to act as coordinators depended on frequent contact and communication with many people. Dealing with so much information and so many people was often stimulating and challenging; but availability was also a problem because it exposed sisters to interruptions.

Interruptions caused a great deal of frustration. They also posed a dilemma for the sisters because on looking at their patterns of work they found that the interrupting contacts and communications were often essential and seldom unnecessary.

The interruption factor seemed to be related to the feeling of being 'in control'. For example, when a sister was particularly busy and felt that she was having difficulty keeping track of ward events, contacts were more likely to be perceived as interruptions. The sisters seemed able to stay in control, as long as they could mentally sort and sift existing information and assimilate new information, as long as they could act on their own work priorities, and as long as it was possible to match the number of nurses and levels of skill to workload requirements. When there were difficulties with one or more of these elements in work, a sister might begin to feel she was losing her grip of the situation.

It also seemed that when the sisters were busy physically and mentally, and when struggling to stay in control, they 'switched off'; that is, they would stop mentally sorting information and selecting high priority work. Instead, they would concentrate on dealing with all-comers in succession, even low priority work, until such time as the pace of work slackened when they could 'switch on' again.

Those sisters who had large numbers of patients, several medical teams, frequent ward rounds, and busy admission and discharge periods seemed to be more often exposed to this kind of pressure; dealing with everyone and everything on the spot could become the customary way of getting through the work. But this way of working which reinforced a sister's availability created a vicious circle, since other people would come to expect that sister should attend to them at once, and might become upset if asked to wait, if redirected to other staff or if asked to make an appointment.

McFarlane (1980), in her *Essays on Nursing*, draws attention to two features of nursing today which she considers 'remarkable'. The first is that the present structure of a nursing team, with its students, staff nurses and ward sister, has shown surprisingly little change since Florence Nightingale's time considering the major alterations which have occurred in job content. The second feature concerns the fact that often the structure of a nursing team is matched 'not so much to meeting patient needs as to an architectural anachronism — the ward'. She suggests that the ward 'is now too large and complex a unit for the management of individualised clinical nursing care' and that 'a patient group manageable by one practitioner as leader of a team of nurses and related to the patients of one physician would be a more rational approach' (p. 20).

In this study it certainly seemed, particularly in the pilot study hospital, that the size of some of the wards in which sisters were working single-handed strongly influenced not only the level of difficulty of their work, but also the number of organisational constraints with which they had to cope and their ability to stay 'in control'. It also seemed that the structure of the team, particularly in terms of whether the ward was designated as a single- or two-sister post, had far-reaching implications, which some sisters were better able to understand than others. One sister remarked that she had too readily assumed that the arrival of a second sister would magically ease her workload and worries. In fact, rather than ease the load, it had radically altered relationships, communications, the nature of responsibility and accountability in the team, and the patterns of patient care management in the ward. The total number of patients and medical teams had not changed, however, and as a result there were still occasions when the volume of information required by each sister remained too great to handle.

The interrelationships between the ways in which sisters work, their ability to cope and organisational factors such as ward size and layout, numbers of patients, number of medical teams and nursing team structure are important and merit closer attention. So far, the models which have been used to examine management issues in nursing seem too simple for the complex reality of ward work.

However, there would seem to be scope for sisters themselves to examine critically the ways in which they use their own time. For example, they could look at their own availability and at the possibility of using appointments. They could note times and activities during which they would prefer not to be interrupted and they could consider how to achieve uninterrupted time. They could also try to recognise and understand self interruption and its relationship to sensory awareness.

Sensory awareness

There were many occasions during observation when it was impossible to record the minute detail of each sister's activities, so rapid was their rate of response to auditory and visual cues. It became apparent that the fragmentation of work, the perceived pressure of work and the amount of self interruption were related to the high level of sensory awareness of the sisters.

The pattern of fragmentation, interruption and responsibility 'often for minute detail' was noted in 1972 by the Committee on Nursing. They stated that it was essential: 'To find some ways of relieving the burdens on ward sisters, and freeing them from day to day minutiae so that they can devote their attention to the overall planning of care in their ward, with more time to exercise their clinical and teaching skills' (p. 42).

The assumption that sisters can, or indeed should, be freed from 'day-to-day minutiae', from fragmentation and interruption has to be questioned. Certainly there were times when the sisters' high level of sensory awareness was more of a hindrance than an asset. For example, it could be difficult to concentrate, to give undivided attention or even to sit still when the mind became too full of detail and 'occult interruptions'. It could be argued, however, that the acute awareness of detail in a ward environment, the ability to pick up and respond to a great many sensory cues, or minutiae, is a vitally important nursing skill — one which may be present in a highly developed form in experienced sisters. If one considers the example given earlier of the sister and the telephone calls (p. 29) it would have been unacceptable if the sister had failed to greet the relatives courteously, as she did; it would also have been professionally unacceptable for a skilled, caring sister to fail to note and respond to the distressed cry of a patient. Ability to deal with this level of minutiae could be considered desirable, essential and part of the nursing art of the sister; freeing a sister from it might be impossible.

In his perceptive account of the role of the sister, Macdonald (1981) recognised that sisters engage in different kinds of work; work 'focused' on the task in hand and 'scanning' or peripheral work through which ward events and the work of others are monitored. In this study, some of the sisters were aware that they combined these two types of work; one sister remarked, that the art lay in being able to give undivided attention to a patient while being able at the same time to store the distracting background information which her eyes and ears were picking up as she concentrated upon the patient.

Macdonald (1981) realised, as did the sisters in this study, that the complexity of a sister's work cannot be captured and understood solely by watching overt activity. By observing, one can detect focused or task work but one cannot unravel fully the mystery of what goes on in a sister's head — the scanning, monitoring, thinking, reflecting and decision-making which are the core elements of her job.

Over a century ago, Florence Nightingale remarked: 'The most important practical lesson that can be given to nurses is to teach them what to observe — how to observe' (1980 p. 88). If sisters gave some thought to that comment and to the following words of Sister Blue and Baroness McFarlane, then it might become possible to identify and describe some of the seemingly hidden core elements of sisters' behaviour and to unravel the mystery of what goes on in sisters' heads.

When Sister Blue talked of difficulties in getting doctors to understand the nursing viewpoint and the nurses' contribution to care, she asked: 'What is it a nurse can see in a patient which isn't necessarily displayed by his pulse, blood pressure or respirations?' In that remark she challenges nurses to identify their observations, the subtle but significant cues which Thomson & Bridge (1981) suggest are the basis of 'the nursing hunch'. And Baroness McFarlane's (1977) comment also challenges nurses to identify the nature of the conventional wisdom of sisters. She says: 'We must all have been impressed at some time in our professional lives by the wisdom of experienced ward sisters.... If we could only catch their wisdom and write it down we would have a rich feast of concepts of nursing practice' (p. 264).

Now that sisters are such a mobile part of the workforce and at a time when an 'experienced' sister may have been only three to five years in that grade, it has become increasingly important to be able to understand the art of sistering and actively to teach others the skills of the job.

Quiet periods
There were times during the on-the-job part of the study when the sisters wished for less pressure or work and complained about having too much to do. However, when the pressure eased and the sisters no longer felt busy, quiet periods were disliked because they were less satisfying and because the sisters did not know what to do with them.

It was suggested that there was an optimum pace and amount of work which was enjoyable and at which the sisters could work well. They liked 'interest' and 'challenge'; 'ill patients' or 'emergency admissions' were welcomed, provided the sisters felt organised and in control and had enough staff to meet patients' needs. When the pace of work lacked momentum, the job became less stimulating and slack periods were bad for morale.

Some of the sisters also lacked ideas and clearly formulated plans for using quiet spells. It was found that rather than change the focus of work or inject pace into it, they would leave the ward early to make up for overtime worked — and they often felt guilty about doing so. And even when ideas and plans did exist, it seemed that the sisters might not develop or use them during their precious spare time. For example, on two occasions, a senior and a junior sister were observed to occupy their time during a quiet period by talking to each other, despite their comments about wishing for more time with patients and more time to teach nurses.

This would suggest that it might not be a sensible policy to wait for quiet periods to introduce changes and new ideas; it might be more realistic to allow developments to take place within the normal untidy pattern and 'optimum' pace of day-to-day work.

Manager and clinician
Among the nine sisters, there seemed to be a wide range of ability to understand the concept of the sister as manager and to interpret the relationship between managerial and clinical components of the job. Comments about management and administration were more often related to site coordination activities; that is, to the organis-

ation of the ward in general rather than to the management of patient care itself. Management concepts were not always understood or regarded as useful and relevant and they were sometimes misinterpreted.

During the on-the-job part of the study, the sisters completed one semantic differential card for each of the concepts Sister as manager, Sister as clinician, Sister as teacher and the Ideal sister, in addition to the six cards for the concept Myself as sister. When the scores for the concepts were compared, it was found that each sister regarded the concept of the Manager as most like the Ideal. This might have been due to the fact that all their professional experience had been within the Salmon era and its management training schemes; in other words, they had lived with the *idea* that sisters were managers. However, although the sisters accepted and used the word manager, they had difficulty applying it within a patient care context and the management function seemed divorced from the clinical and teaching components of the job. For example, Sister Grey saw herself as least like the ideal (the manager) and most like the clinician and teacher, and it was striking that in her ward it had been decided that the senior sister would deal with 'the administration and office work' while Sister Grey would deal with 'the teaching and the clinical work'.

Administrative 'chores'
It is sometimes assumed that administrative tasks and office work are regarded by sisters as chores and that ward clerks should help by relieving sisters of such work. However, some of the comments about administration showed that these assumptions should be questioned, as they oversimplify the complex nature of this part of a sister's work. The help of the ward clerk in dealing with clerical work and the telephone was certainly valued but it was not necessarily felt to reduce a sister's workload; the ward clerk's work had to be planned and coordinated and she could be yet another source of interruption. Also, work delegated to a ward clerk would not necessarily be regarded simply as a chore. Dealing with a patient's admission, for example, involved more than just clerical work; it contained essential nursing elements. One sister felt that it was important to greet new patients as soon as possible after their arrival in the ward, not only out of courtesy and concern for good relationship, but also to observe each one and make an early nursing assessment. This sister also happened to enjoy clerical work and she often shared the paper work with the ward clerk by combining aspects of documentation with her assessment observations.

The more perceptive sisters recognised that it was important to retain nursing elements within work which might otherwise be labelled by onlookers as 'non-nursing'. These sisters underlined the need to analyse tasks and to identify the nursing essentials in them lest they be taken over by others. The sister's comments about the attractions of a plated-meal and waitress service suggest that some sisters might not be alert enough to important nursing skills inherent in routine day-to-day work (p. 87).

The most senior sister suspected that there had been a gradual but steady rise in the volume of administrative and paper work in her ward, a trend which she attributed to increased turnover of patients. It was interesting, however, that she had no facts about bed occupancy over the years; she only had 'hunches' that the situation was changing. It seemed as though the sisters worked in an information vacuum, surrounded by ungathered facts which might have provided the evidence to support or refute their hunches; evidence which could have helped the sisters to carry out informed evaluation of nursing care management in their wards.

Direct nursing care
As far as direct contact with patients was concerned, it seemed that the sisters needed some involvement in 'basic care' to maintain job satisfaction and self esteem. Contact was also recognised, to varying extents, as being essential to the assessment and planning of patient care, to the supervision and teaching of learners and to the maintenance of clinical expertise.

Most of the sisters had experienced some conflict between the clinical, managerial and teaching functions of the role and for various reasons most wanted to have more contact with patients. However, the sister who spent least time in direct patient care and most time on administration was satisfied with the distribution of her time and energies between these three functions.

The care received by the patients in each ward was not examined in this study, therefore it was not possible to say whether the different interpretations of the sister's role and the sisters' varying patterns of work had any influence upon the patients themselves. The possible relationships between the sister's concept of her role, her systems of care management and the quality of care the patients receive still needs to be examined. Meantime, however, the current interest in the process of nursing might bring into focus the clinical management role of the sister and might help to clarify the close interrelationship between the three components of the job.

Teacher

Each sister accepted that she had a teaching function, but some were unclear about their teaching responsibilities and all felt that preparation for this part of the role had been inadequate.

The problems identified were lack of time for teaching, lack of a knowledge base and teaching skills, lack of confidence in teaching ability, lack of expert specialist help with teaching, and inability to assess learner needs and performance.

Confirmation of Lelean's (1973) finding that sisters spend little time with the most junior learners is important and worrying, if it is accepted that sisters have a special contribution to make towards teaching, assessing and supporting those in the early stages of training. But what is the special contribution of the sister and to whom should it be directed? It could be argued, for example, that it might be more sensible for a sister to invest time in observing, assessing and teaching senior rather than junior learners in view of the fact that seniors often have to undertake, in a sister's absence, the more complex interpersonal, problem-solving and decision-making elements in her work.

To help answer these questions, there is now evidence from several studies, undertaken during the 1970s, regarding the special part which sisters play in relation to the ward-based teaching and learning of all students. For example, the work of Fretwell (1980), Orton (1981), Marson (1981) and Ogier (1982) has helped to explain the relationship between a sister and the type of learning climate which exists in a ward in terms of the things that a sister actually needs to *do* as teacher and the kind of person the sister needs to *be* in order to facilitate learning. Their work shows clearly that there is a great deal more to teaching than didactic instruction or telling. It seems that in addition to considerable commitment to and active involvement in teaching, a sister needs high-level interpersonal skills and awareness of her own behaviour and attitudes in order to be an effective teacher and to create a good climate for learning (p. 7).

In this study, the sisters' comments and the observed fragmentation of work together suggested that reliance on 'formal' teaching which requires longer, uninterrupted periods of time might not be the most practical method for sisters to use. What they seemed to need was ability to use effectively their brief contacts with learners. Some of the sisters did realise that such contacts, anywhere in the ward, even the kitchen, could provide valuable teaching–learning opportunities. However, as the most experienced sister recognised, the phrase 'teaching by example' needs to be carefully examined, and the meaning of the phrase 'the teachable moment' needs to be explored if brief teaching–learning opportunities are to be used well. Being available to learners can provide them with chances to observe a sister at work; but it does not guarantee that the learner perceives the sister as approachable or available to answer questions, even if she does know the questions to ask. Simply being with sister does not guarantee that learning will occur. Contact between a sister and a junior nurse, who may seldom have spoken to each other, might be no more than an anxious moment for the learner. Without help, a learner will possibly not be able to observe, interpret and understand the nursing essentials in the things she does and sees.

In order to make effective use of teachable moments, sisters need to know the learners' needs, to recognise the learning opportunities available in their wards, and be able to match the two.

In a course designed to help sisters with teaching methods, Ford and his colleagues (1979) found that in addition to lack of knowledge about basic teaching principles, and difficulties with recognising learning situations, there were particular problems with setting teaching objectives and with lack of in-depth knowledge. All these problems were expressed in this study and it also seemed that some sisters were unclear about what they most needed to know in terms of the nursing knowledge which was relevant to the clinical practice available in their own wards. There was confusion between nursing-related and medicine-related knowledge and more anxiety about being out of touch and about keeping up to date with the latter than the former. Clearly it was important for the sisters to know about new drugs and about those changes in the treatments and techniques of doctors which had direct implications for their work. However, it was equally important that they should be aware of, and be discussing with their teams, new information about nursing practice; for example, concerning skin care, bowel care, mouth care, food intake, and pre- and postoperative nursing care (Macleod Clark & Hockey 1979). With the exception of some pilot study sisters, there seemed to be little awareness of the fact that 'not knowing about' these aspects of nursing work could have important care, comfort and safety implications for their patients.

The final teaching problems concerned lack of expert help and assessment of learners. In an experiment which aimed to integrate nursing theory and practice, it was found that 70 per cent of the trained staff involved in the study did not know whether the students had had the relevant theoretical preparation for the work required in their wards (Alexander 1983). Some of the nine sisters in this study remarked that they would have benefited from having more information about each learner as she arrived and for this reason would have welcomed closer liaison with their colleagues in education.

More help with clinical teaching or more effective use of the existing help would also have been welcomed. In one ward, however, the clinical teacher had been integrated successfully into the ward team and a planned teaching programme had been developed jointly by all the registered nurses involved, the staff nurses, the clinical teacher and the ward sisters.

It is possible that many sisters might echo the telling comment of one in this study, that she did not 'know' the student when the time came to write her assessment. However, as Sister Blue showed, the problem of assessment can be tackled by asking questions about what a nurse needs to know and about the kinds of clinical experience and special expertise available in a ward. When these questions had not been answered, or indeed even asked, a diffuse anxiety seemed to surround 'how the student was getting on in the ward'. Bendall (1976), discussing 'learning for reality' said that 'the central core of nurse training and education lies in the reality of clinical patient care'. The remarks of the nine sisters would suggest, however, that they need help to acquire teaching skills and to understand their influence upon ward learning. Unless they receive more effective teaching support from others, it may be difficult for learners to benefit fully from a sister's expertise and to understand satisfactorily and learn about the reality of clinical patient care.

Conflict

The sisters showed that the demands of their role created strain and conflict — conflict between roles, conflict within the role and self-role conflict.

Self-expectations in some cases seemed to be extremely high and were probably unrealistic considering the sisters' circumstances. The sister who perceived herself as being in a situation where 'everybody expects you to do everything' was trying to cope with several organisational difficulties which included mixed specialty nursing in a large ward with an awkward layout, and having 'to battle' to communicate with four medical teams each with its own specialist interests. She felt overwhelmed by the demands of the job. Her morale seemed low and she talked of being dispirited and of feeling that she was 'failing'. It seemed significant that this sister's greatest problem was getting the nursing officer to understand the ward, and clearly she did not feel at the time that she was getting the kind of personal support which she needed. In order to cope, she worked overtime and took work home, but she resented the fact that the job encroached upon her social life. She was also worried about the implications of the shorter working week, and she could not see how she would be able to cope with what seemed to be ever-increasing work demands within shorter periods of time.

Sometimes the nature of conflict did not seem to be understood; the actual expectations of various role-set members were not always known and attempts at discovering others' expectations might not have been made. For example, the care-versus-cure dilemma caused some of the sisters considerable anxiety and conflict but not all of them had attempted to discuss this important inter-professional issue with their colleagues. As a result, it seemed that assumptions about others' expectations were being made; work difficulties tended to be oversimplified and the sisters sometimes internalised the blame for problems, perceiving them as 'my fault'. The difficulties with unit meetings illustrated these points. The sisters complied with the perceived expectations — and possibly the actual expectations — of the nursing officer that they should go to all unit meetings, despite having prior appointments and despite their own professional judgement that staff left in the ward were not competent enough to deal with work in their absence.

Sister Grey's ward round morning illustrated several types of conflict and strain (p. 39). There was the conflict of meeting self-expectations about quantity of work at the expense of ideals about 'quality' of work; there was conflict with the perceived expectations of doctors; there was conflict between work and family when work demands encroached on personal time; and Sister Grey also experienced overload and conflict between work priorities.

The examples of conflict suggest that sisters and their colleagues in the ward team need to examine their personal and professional value systems. Studying the causes and effects of conflict could serve the interests of the professional growth and job satisfaction of sisters as well as the interests of patient care itself.

The nursing officer
This small sample of sisters experienced difficulties across the whole range of nursing officer functions as they were originally envisaged by the Salmon Committee, and their comments would seem to support the views of the Royal Commission on the National Health Service (1979) that the original concept of the nursing officer should be developed.

The sisters did differ in their expectations of the nursing officer.

Not all were unhappy about existing relationships. One was content simply that the nursing officer did not 'interfere' but others were clearly dissatisfied with her contribution to the ward. Communications were sometimes poor, mutual expectations unclear and the relationship unsupportive. The sisters outlined several aspects of work in which they would have valued more effective help from their nursing officer; with certain aspects, some sisters seemed to perceive that they were getting no help at all.

Management of resources
Fluctuations in workload and staffing levels were a regular problem. The sisters would have welcomed facts and feedback about changing trends in staffing, dependency, workload and bed occupancy, in addition to better short-term advice and help on how to deal with hour by hour staffing–workload imbalances.

Clinical and teaching work
The nursing officer was perceived as being 'out of touch' and as having forgotten about the reality and 'stresses' of ward work. As a result, the sisters felt that they could not draw on her expertise to give specialist advice on clinical matters, to teach learners or to help analyse clinical problems and monitor standards of care. It seemed that some more active form of participation in the management and delivery of care would have helped restore the nursing officers' credibility in the eyes of the sisters. However, some of the sisters did realise that this might 'tread on their toes'. They acknowledged that any new relationships in clinical care management would need to be carefully negotiated and sensitively handled and would need to take into account the *actual* level of the nursing officer's clinical expertise.

Staff appraisal and development
The sisters felt that they could have been given more help with the assessment and counselling of their team especially when problems arose. It was disturbing that one sister, anxious about a member of staff's alcohol problem, should have perceived that 'nothing could be done' and that she should have been left hoping that the situation would resolve itself.

It also seemed that the sisters were given little feedback about their own performance and some would have welcomed an opportunity to step aside and take stock of their own work.

Learning the job

All sisters seemed to feel that the most useful ways of learning the role were by watching and listening to the role model and by being 'left to get on with it'. Off-the-job management courses were regarded as being of limited value and some of their content inappropriate or too abstract to relate to ward work.

Some sisters remarked that when they were staff nurses, they had been aware of the status or 'place' of the sister but they had not understood the duties and responsibilities of the role nor how to deal with them. The process of discovering about the range of responsibilities had been slow and sometimes painful. 'Hit and miss' learning had proved to be inefficient and costly to both the sisters and to patient care and it seemed that each sister might meet the same difficulties and make the same mistakes as her predecessors. Supposedly reassuring remarks about 'taking at least a year to get into the job' had done little to lessen feelings of insecurity or to help sisters to cope with other people's altered expectations when status changed suddenly from staff nurse to sister.

It has long been recognised that the attitudes, values and behaviour of sisters do influence learners and staff nurses, some of whom in time become sisters or role models themselves. Through watching a sister at work, a nurse may identify with and imitate the behaviour of the sister whom she perceives as 'good'.

Role modelling can be a potent force in learning but it has its problems. For example, role models may display desirable or undesirable behaviour; they may perpetuate outdated practice and attitudes and it cannot be assumed that staff nurses will model themselves on 'good' sisters.

The labelling of a sister as 'good' may be based on 'liking' or 'respect' for her as a person, rather than on clearly identified criteria of desirable or effective behaviour and appropriate attitudes. There would seem to be an urgent need to identify the 'good' role model.

A sister's level of awareness of her own attitudes, values and behaviour and her ability to talk about her job might be further problems with role modelling. Some of the sisters in this study seemed to be unclear about certain aspects of their own behaviour; they found it difficult to look objectively at their work and to 'put the job into words'.

What seems to be needed is a more efficient on-the-job training system based upon 'good' sisters acting as role models; sisters who have a high level of self-awareness of their own attitudes and behaviour, who are able not only to demonstrate but also to talk about and explain the nature of the job and who are given support to carry out their training function. A number of experimental ward-based training schemes are currently being developed and evaluated in Britain (Slack 1981, Farnish 1982).

There is probably some truth in the suggestion that a sister cannot know whether a day is good or bad and how to deal with it, until she has experienced a range of good and bad days and dealt with them; only after a period of time in a ward can past and present experience be put into perspective. But it may be that the phrase 'learning the job through experience' is an example of a ritual remark which has masked a basic problem of failure to define roles and failure to teach trainee sisters to deal effectively with the complex responsibilities of the job.

Traditional role learning by slow absorption and by long experience is neither efficient nor realistic at a time when greater frequency of staff turnover has reduced the time available for observing the model. To make a role clear to others, expectations must be communicated. If the sister is herself unclear about her role, then her staff nurses may also be confused. Banton's (1965) definition of the poor supervisor may be uncomfortably apt for some sisters:

> The poor supervisor is the man who fails to make clear to his subordinates what is expected of them.... The poor supervisor does not communicate his expectations because he has never been taught to think explicitly about the role he has to play; probably he has learned his tasks by watching others and is inclined to take the organisational pattern for granted. (p. 211)

Continuing education

The Scottish report (1981) on continuing education for the nursing profession firmly challenges the belief that the basic preparation for nursing is sufficient for a lifetime of practice. It also expresses concern about the low level of provision of planned educational opportunities for nurses at their place of work and throughout their working lives.

The report suggests that:

- All practitioners need regular updating of their knowledge and skills in order to maintain their clinical expertise and professional awareness.
- There should be an identifiable programme of continuing edu-

cation opportunities within and outwith the nurse's place of
work

• On-the-job elements of continuing education should be closely
related to an effective system of staff appraisal and staff development which will identify the potential strengths and the training
needs of all nurses

The report also points out that the success of continuing education ventures will depend not only on effective staff appraisal,
on realistic resource allocation of finance and manpower, and on
close collaboration between nurse managers and education staff,
but also on the extent to which individual nurses accept responsibility for keeping themselves up to date and using the resources
available.

Some of the sisters in this study were actively involved in continuing education. They read and they sought information from a
wide range of sources in order to update their knowledge and to
keep abreast of changes and developments in their own and other
professions; and they undertook these activities on their own initiative. Other sisters, however, were not motivated towards keeping
themselves up to date or towards review of clinical practice and
ward management, and for these sisters a change of attitudes and
more information about the need for continuing education would
have been essential.

Change
Awareness of the need for change and innovation varied considerably. The sisters who had ideas and who were motivated to innovate outlined several difficulties which they had met in their
attempts to plan and negotiate change and to gain acceptance for
their ideas.

It had been difficult to find time in the ward during working
hours to think about and plan for change. Some sisters did not have
a room of their own to which they could go for peace and quiet;
lack of peace and privacy for reflection, and for other aspects of
work such as interviewing relatives, was a major problem.

In order to get uninterrupted time during working hours the sisters would have had to be prepared to leave their wards and seek a
quiet place elsewhere within or outwith the hospital, or they might
have had to find some way of reducing their availability and ensur-
ing privacy within the ward area. One sister in the study indicated
that she was 'not available' by locking her office door, another sister
changed out of her uniform.

It is sometimes suggested that sisters should be willing to devote some of their own time to work activities in the interest of their own professional development. However, the assumption that sisters should give personal time to professional matters has to be treated with caution. Some of the sisters were willing but simply not able to do so for various reasons. One sister said that often she was just too tired physically and emotionally at the end of a day's work to start thinking and planning; another sister found that her personal time was fully occupied with her home commitments, which included caring for children and elderly relatives.

It seemed that the sisters, and possibly their nurse managers, needed to come to terms with the idea that sitting down thinking, or reading or discussing ideas with others were legitimate parts of professional activity during working hours.

Some sisters found that it had taken time and perseverance to discuss an idea with the many people directly and indirectly involved in proposed change. Ideas had to be 'sold', and the co-operation of staff gained; the levels of interest of staff, their motivation and commitment had to be assessed and could vary. Comparatively minor changes could take months or even years to introduce and evaluate, and it could be extremely difficult to eradicate well-established outdated practice. Change could also be perceived as a threat to a sister's popularity, and waiting for 'spare moments' to introduce change was found to be unsatisfactory because such moments seldom occurred or were not used effectively.

It also seemed that a sister might feel constrained by the nursing officer and might not perceive herself as free to initiate ideas; alternatively, change initiated by senior management could be perceived as an unwanted imposition. Even when a sister was highly motivated towards experimenting with ideas, the introduction of change into the complex and unstable environment of a ward might be avoided because of the risk of increasing the complexity, adding to the instability, and upsetting routine and relationships. It could be easier to adhere to well-established routine and to 'keep the system working', especially when under pressure.

Some sisters seemed to welcome the idea of discussing problems and ideas for change with others, such as their peers or the nursing officer. The sister who enjoyed problem solving regarded her nursing officer as a 'sounding board', as someone with whom ideas could be shared, problems discussed and objectives set. Other sisters clearly would have required help to analyse problems, to set long and short-term objectives for change, and to understand the organisational constraints which so easily seemed to sabotage the best-laid schemes for innovation.

Isolation

Some sisters were aware of a need to learn from each other; others were not, and were happy in their isolation. Those sisters who acknowledged their own expertise and the expertise of their colleagues felt that it should be possible to develop in a structured way the exchange of professional information — a 'neglected' area. Casual contact over meals or the telephone was valuable and often provided moral support and a chance to talk about problems, but some sisters wanted more than this. They wanted to share ideas, skills and knowledge, and the most senior sister would have welcomed a system of peer review of job performance.

In order to meet other colleagues, however, the sisters would have had to overcome the difficulties of getting out of their ward areas. Lack of staff considered competent to deal with a sister's delegated work in her absence was an obvious reason for reluctance to leave and discomfort when out of the ward. But even when competent staff were available, some sisters seemed guilty and vaguely uneasy about the idea of leaving the ward, so accustomed had they become to being within its four walls for most of each shift.

If such difficulties could be overcome, there might be considerable scope for developing, on a unit or hospital basis, peer review and support groups for sisters.

The inevitability of problems

Throughout the study, during the interviews and in conversations with the sisters one theme kept recurring — the inevitability of problems.

Considering the complex nature of the job, its organisational constraints and the lingering influences of history and tradition within the profession, the sisters were probably accurate in their assessment that certain aspects of the job are inevitable; aspects such as interruptions, conflicts of opinion with medical colleagues, tiredness, being 'further away from patients' and being less involved in giving direct care. What must be questioned, however, is the assumption that 'nothing can be done' about these and other aspects of the job when they are perceived as problems.

It was encouraging that some sisters were willing to analyse and to attempt to solve problems. Some had a great deal of insight into the factors which influenced their perceptions of their work difficulties, and some had both sought and received help in dealing with them.

Nevertheless, the fatalism of other sisters about the insoluble nature of their problems was disturbing. Their fatalism and their perceived lack of support in the face of work difficulties are a challenge to the profession.

References

Foreword

Fretwell J E 1980 An enquiry into the ward learning environment. Occasional Papers. Nursing Times 76 (26): 69–75

Knowles H P, Saxberg B O 1971 Personality and leadership behaviour. Addison-Wesley, Cambridge, Mass., p 36

Ogier M E 1982 An ideal sister? Royal College of Nursing, London

Orton H D 1981 Ward learning climate and student nurse response. Occasional Papers. Nursing Times 77(23): 65–68

Pembrey S 1980 The ward sister — key to nursing. Royal College of Nursing, London

Redfern S J 1981 Hospital sisters — their job attitudes and occupational stability. Royal College of Nursing, London

Chapter 1

Abel-Smith B 1960 A history of the nursing profession. Heinemann, London

Anderson E R 1973 The role of the nurse. Royal College of Nursing, London

Bendall E 1976 Learning for reality. Journal of Advanced Nursing 1: 3–9

British Medical Journal 1974 Leading article. British Medical Journal iv

British Medical Journal 1981 Doctors and nurses. Editorial. British Medical Journal 283: 683–684

Cartwright A 1964 Human relations and hospital care. Routledge & Kegan Paul, London

Cortazzi D, Roote S 1975 Illuminative incident analysis. McGraw-Hill, Maidenhead

Davies J 1972 A study of hospital management training in its organisational context. Centre for Business Research, University of Manchester

Department of Health and Social Security 1968 Report of a Committee of the Central Health Services Council: Relieving nurses of non-nursing duties in general and maternity hospitals (Farrer Report). HMSO, London

Department of Health and Social Security 1972 Report of the Committee on Nursing (Briggs Report) Cmnd 5115. HMSO, London

Elliott M, Fisher R 1979 Management audit — the Exeter method. Occasional Paper. Nursing Times 75(22): 89–92

Fretwell J E 1980 An inquiry into the ward learning environment. Occasional Paper. Nursing Times 76(16): 69–75

Gray A, Smail R 1981 A review of trends in the Scottish hospital nursing labour force. Health Economics Research Unit, Aberdeen University

Greater Glasgow Health Board 1975 Ruchill Hospital: A Report to the Greater Glasgow Health Board. Glasgow

Heyman B, Shaw M 1980 Nurses' perceptions of the British hospital nursing officer. Journal of Advanced Nursing 5: 613–623

Hockey L 1976 Women in nursing. Hodder & Stoughton, London

Huczynski A 1977 Nursing management audit: the reaction of users. Journal of Advanced Nursing 2: 521–531

Jenkinson V M 1965 The ward sister in relation to administration and research. International Journal of Nursing Studies 2: 105–113

Jones D, Crossley-Holland C, Matus T 1981 The role of the nursing officer. DHSS, London

King's Fund Project Report 1981 Training ward for ward sisters. King's Fund Centre, London

Lelean S R 1973 Ready for report nurse? Royal College of Nursing, London

McFarlane J K 1976 A charter for caring. Journal of Advanced Nursing 1: 187–196

McFarlane J 1980 Essays on nursing. King's Fund Centre, London

McGhee A 1961 The patient's attitude to nursing care. E & S Livingstone, Edinburgh

MacGuire J M 1961 From student to nurse. Part 1: The induction period. Oxford Area Nurse Training Committee

Mackenzie J 1973 A ward sister's impressions of university students. Unpublished report from a conference of the Association of Integrated and Degree Courses in Nursing

Ministry of Health and Scottish Home and Health Department 1966 Report of the Committee on Senior Nursing Staff Structure (Salmon Report). HMSO, London

Orton H D 1981 Ward learning climate and student nurse response. Occasional Paper. Nursing Times 77(17): 65–68

Pembrey S 1980 The ward sister — key to nursing. Royal College of Nursing, London

Redfern S J 1981 Hospital sisters. Royal College of Nursing, London

Revans R W 1964 Standards for morale, cause and effect in hospitals. Nuffield Provincial Hospitals Trust. Oxford University Press, Oxford

Royal Commission on the National Health Service 1979 Cmnd 7615. HMSO, London

Royal Infirmary of Edinburgh, Minute Book of Nursing Committee 1915–1924

Royal Infirmary of Edinburgh, Minute Book of Nursing Committee 1924–1930

Rules and Regulations of the Royal Infirmary of Edinburgh 1881 Crawford & McCabe, Edinburgh

Salmon versus the doctors 1974 Nursing Times 70(9): 296–297

The Scotsman 1975 News items, February 1, March 18, March 25

Tolliday H 1972 Defining the nurse's role. Occasional Paper. Nursing Times 68(14): 53–56

Toman J P 1977 Health service management training. Nursing Times 73(27): 1041–1043

Wall T, Hespe G 1972 The attitudes of nurses towards the Salmon structure. Occasional Paper. Nursing Times 68: 105–108

Wells T 1980 Problems in geriatric nursing care. Churchill Livingstone, Edinburgh

White D, Frawley A 1975 Partnership in management development. Occasional Paper. Nursing Times 71(33): 81–84

Williams D, Message M 1969 Management courses for senior nursing staff. International Nurses Review 16: 329–337

Chapter 2

Banton M 1965 Roles. An introduction to the study of social relations. Tavistock Publications, London

Benne K, Bennis W 1959 Role confusion and conflict in nursing. The role of the professional nurse. American Journal of Nursing 59(2): 196–198

Boulding K 1964 Two principles of conflict. In: Kahn R, Boulding E (eds) Power and conflict in organisations. Tavistock Publications, London

Chapman C M 1976 The use of sociological theories and models in nursing. Journal of Advanced Nursing 1: 111–127

Coser L A 1967 Continuities in the study of social conflict. Free Press, New York

Davies J 1972 A study of hospital management training in its organisational context. Centre for Business Research, University of Manchester

Hansen A, Upshaw H 1962 Evaluation within the context of role analysis. Nursing Research 11(3): 144–150

Kahn R, Wolfe D 1964 Role conflict in organisations. In: Kahn R, Boulding E (eds) Power and conflict in organisations. Tavistock Publications, London

Kahn R L, Wolfe D M, Quinn R P, Snoek J D, Rosenthal R A 1964 Organizational stress: studies in role conflict and ambiguity. Wiley, New York

McFarlane J K 1977 Developing a theory of nursing: the relation of theory to practice, education and research. Journal of Advanced Nursing 2: 261–270

Menzies I 1960 A case study in the functioning of social systems as a defence against anxiety. Human Relations 13: 95–121

Merton R K 1957a Social theory and social structure. Free Press, Glencoe, Illinois

Merton R K 1957b The role-set: problems in sociological theory. British Journal of Sociology 8: 106–120

Snoek J D 1966 Role strain in diversified role sets. American Journal of Sociology 71(4): 363–372

Wolfe D, Snoek J 1962 A study of tensions and adjustment under role conflict. Journal of Social Issues 18: 121

Chapter 3

Goddard H A 1953 The work of nurses in hospital wards. Nuffield Provincial Hospitals Trust, London

Hall D U 1978 'What nurse don't see, she don't worry about' or The use of observation in hospital research. Occasional Paper. Nursing Times 74(34): 137–140

Heise D 1969 Some methodological issues in semantic differential research. Psychological Bulletin 72(6): 406–422

Kerlinger F N 1965 Foundations of behavioural research. Holt, Rinehart & Winston, London

Osgood C E, Suci G J, Tannenbaum F H 1957 The measurement of meaning. University of Illinois Press, Urbana

Pembrey S 1980 The ward sister — key to nursing. Royal College of Nursing, London

Runciman P J 1980 Ward sisters' perceptions of problems in their work role. M. Phil Thesis, University of Edinburgh

Treece E W, Treece J W 1977 Elements of research in nursing, 2nd edn. C V Mosby, St Louis

Warr P B, Knapper C 1968 The perception of people and events. Wiley, London

Watson P J 1979 Studying work. Nursing Times 75(20): 81–84

Chapter 5

Lelean S R 1973 Ready for report nurse? Royal College of Nursing, London

Pembrey S 1980 The ward sister — key to nursing. Royal College of Nursing, London

Siegel S 1956 Non-parametric statistics for the behavioural sciences. McGraw-Hill, New York

Chapter 6

Alexander M 1983 Learning to nurse: integrating theory and practice. Churchill Livingstone, Edinburgh

Banton M 1965 Roles. An introduction to the study of social relations. Tavistock Publications, London

Bendall E 1976 Learning for reality. Journal of Advanced Nursing 1: 3–9

Continuing education for the nursing profession in Scotland 1981 Report of a working party on continuing education and professional development for nurses, midwives and health visitors. Edinburgh

Department of Health and Social Security 1972 Report of the Committee on Nursing (Briggs Report). Cmnd 5115. HMSO, London

Farnish S 1982 'Thrown in at the deep end'. Nursing Times 78(10): 404–405

Fretwell J E 1980 An inquiry into the ward learning environment. Occasional Paper. Nursing Times 76(16): 69–75

Ford J, Redmond I, Roach F 1979 A pilot course on ward teaching methods. Occasional Paper. Nursing Times 75(3): 13–16

Lelean S R 1973 Ready for report nurse? Royal College of Nursing, London

Macdonald I 1981 Role of the ward sister. Health and Social Service Journal 91: 565–569

McFarlane J K 1977 Developing a theory of nursing: the relation of theory to practice, education and research. Journal of Advanced Nursing 2: 261–270

McFarlane J 1980 Essays on nursing. King's Fund Centre, London

Macleod Clark J, Hockey L 1979 Research for nursing: a guide for the enquiring nurse. HM+M Publishers, Aylesbury

Marson S N 1981 Ward teaching skills — an investigation into the behavioural characteristics of effective ward teachers. M. Phil Thesis, Sheffield City Polytechnic

Nightingale F 1980 Notes on nursing. Churchill Livingstone, Edinburgh.

Ogier M 1982 An ideal sister? Royal College of Nursing, London

Orton H D 1981 Ward learning climate and student nurse response. Occasional Paper. Nursing Times 77(17): 65–68

Royal Commission on the National Health Service 1979 Cmnd 7615. HMSO, London

Slack P 1981 Ward sister training. Nursing Times 77(2): 53

Thomson B, Bridge W 1981 Teaching patient care. Guidance for the practising nurse. HM+M Publishers, Aylesbury

Further reading

Broadley M E 1980 Patients come first. Nursing at 'The London' between the two world wars. The London Hospital Special Trustees, London

Department of Health and Social Security and Welsh Office 1976 Report of a Committee of the Central Health Services Council: The organisation of the in-patient's day. HMSO, London

Evers H 1982 Key issues in nursing practice: ward management-1; ward management-2. Occasional Papers. Nursing Times 78(6 & 7): 21–24; 25–26

Fretwell J E 1980 Hospital ward routine — friend or foe? Journal of Advanced Nursing 5: 625–636

Hunt C D 1980 A course for sisters and charge nurses. Nursing Times 76: 2145–2146

Hyde White H 1978 Do-it-yourself in-service training. Nursing Times 74(51): 2117–2118

Luckes E 1886 Hospital sisters and their duties. Scientific Press, London

Moores B, Moult A 1979 Patterns of nurse activity. Journal of Advanced Nursing 4: 137–149

Oppenheim A N 1966 Questionnaire design and attitude measurement. Heinemann, London

Pembrey S 1981 Voice of the ward sister. Nursing Focus 2(7): 218–219

Royal College of Nursing 1981 Towards standards — a discussion document. RCN, London

Scottish Home and Health Department 1974 Review of the senior nursing staff structure. Edinburgh

Sheahan J 1978 Ward sister — manager, nurse, or teacher? Nursing Mirror 146(20): 18–21

Smith J P 1977 The unit nursing officer: manager of nursing care. Journal of Advanced Nursing 2: 571–588

Smyth M 1980 Site-base first-line management training. Nursing Times 76: 2143–2144

Stapleton M 1982 Update, top-ranking. Nursing Mirror 154(12): 38–40

Appendix 1

Activity code list

Activity	Code
Primary care—basic and technical	10
Observing patient	12
Medicines	13
Sister's ward round	14
Talking with patient	15
Checking charts	16
Serving/distributing meals	17
Formal report to/from nurses	20
Receiving work report from nurses	21
Prescribing work—ad hoc order	22
Teaching	24
Talking with nurse	25
Doctor's ward round	31
Talking with doctor	35
Interaction with unit nursing officer	40
Interaction with other senior nursing staff	41
Interaction with ward clerk	42
Interaction with clinical teacher	43
Interaction with friends and relatives of patients	44
Interaction with other hospital staff	46
Interaction with domestics	47
Interaction with physiotherapist	48
Making/receiving phone calls	60
Writing/reading Kardex	61
Looking for people or equipment	62
Writing nursing orders	63
Attending unit meeting	64
General administration	66
Clearing away equipment	67
Absent from ward on official duties	69
Personal time	70
Hand washing	75
Walking time	76
Unskilled work	80
Talking to the observer	90
Unidentified activity	99

Appendix 2

Activity fragmentation: number and percentage of observations in each time category

Number of observations

Duration of activity	Sister Gold	Green	Grey	Brown	White	Black	Pink
<1 min	396	616	898	522	504	783	763
1–<2 min	382	314	455	352	324	367	411
2–<5 min	145	152	166	183	157	158	155
5–<10 min	48	30	38	48	49	33	28
10 min and over	16	23	8	17	22	17	15
Total	987	1135	1565	1122	1056	1358	1372

Percentage of observations

Duration of activity	Sister Gold	Green	Grey	Brown	White	Black	Pink
<1 min	40.1	54.3	57.4	46.5	47.7	57.6	55.6
1–<2 min	38.7	27.7	29.1	31.4	30.7	27.0	30.0
2–<5 min	14.7	13.4	10.6	16.3	14.9	11.6	11.3
5–<10 min	4.9	2.6	2.4	4.3	4.6	2.8	2.0
10 min and over	1.6	2.0	0.5	1.5	2.1	1.0	1.1
Total	100.0%	100.0%	100.0%	100.0%	100.0%	100.0%	100.0%

Appendix 3

The 25 problem statements: each sister's rank order and rating

Having enough contact with the patients
Statement rank order = 1. Rank total = 48.

	Sister Blue*	Red*	Gold	Green	Grey	Brown	White	Black	Pink
Rank order	1	5	2	5	2	7	14	4	8
Rating	+++++	++++	+++++	++++	+++++	+++	++	++++	+++

Finding time to talk with the patients in a leisurely way
Statement rank order = 2. Rank Total = 51.

	Sister Blue*	Red*	Gold	Green	Grey	Brown	White	Black	Pink
Rank order	2	7	8	4	7	3	4	6	10
Rating	+++++	++++	++++	++++	+++	+++++	++++	+++	+++

Being interrupted so often
Statement rank order = tied rank 3.5. Rank total = 57.

	Sister Blue*	Red*	Gold	Green	Grey	Brown	White	Black	Pink
Rank order	8	1	6	3	23	1	7	7	1
Rating	++++	+++++	++++	+++++	+	+++++	+++	+++	+++++

Teaching the student nurses
Statement rank order = tied rank 3.5. Rank total = 57.

	Sister Blue*	Red*	Gold	Green	Grey	Brown	White	Black	Pink
Rank order	4	16	4	2	6	2	9	2	12
Rating	+++++	++	+++++	+++++	+++	+++++	+++	++++	++

*not observed

Having enough contact with the student nurses
Statement rank order = 5. Rank total = 69.

	Sister Blue*	Red*	Gold	Green	Grey	Brown	White	Black	Pink
Rank order	6	15	3	1	8	6	12	1	17
Rating	+++++	++	+++++	+++++	++	++++	++	+++++	++ -

Meeting the demands of so many people
Statement rank order = 6. Rank total = 83.

	Sister Blue*	Red*	Gold	Green	Grey	Brown	White	Black	Pink
Rank order	7	3	17	16	3	5	15	12	5
Rating	++++	+++++	++	++	++++	++++	++	++	++++

Being available to everyone while on duty
Statement rank order = 7. Rank total = 92.

	Sister Blue*	Red*	Gold	Green	Grey	Brown	White	Black	Pink
Rank order	9	9	12	9	5	13	20	11	4
Rating	++++	+++	+++	+++	+++	+	+	++	++++

Having too much to do each day
Statement rank order = tied rank 8.5. Rank total = 95.

	Sister Blue*	Red*	Gold	Green	Grey	Brown	White	Black	Pink
Rank order	14	6	5	18	13	12	1	13	13
Rating	+++	++++	++++	++	+	++	+++++	++	++

Finding out whether the work is being done
Statement rank order = tied rank 8.5. Rank total = 95.

	Sister Blue*	Red*	Gold	Green	Grey	Brown	White	Black	Pink
Rank order	3	4	18	13	4	11	19	3	20
Rating	+++++	++++	++	+++	+++	++	+	++++	+

*not observed

Doing basic nursing care
Statement rank order = 10. Rank total = 101.

	Sister Blue*	Red*	Gold	Green	Grey	Brown	White	Black	Pink
Rank order	5	14	7	8	1	14	24	25	3
Rating	+++++	++	++++	+++	+++++	+	+	+	++++

Getting the nursing officer to understand the ward
Statement rank order = 11. Rank total = 109.

	Sister Blue*	Red*	Gold	Green	Grey	Brown	White	Black	Pink
Rank order	11	8	1	19	20	18	18	8	6
Rating	++++	+++	+++++	++	+	+	++	+++	++++

Feeling tired
Statement rank order = 12. Rank total = 123.

	Sister Blue*	Red*	Gold	Green	Grey	Brown	White	Black	Pink
Rank order	12	20	10	21	25	23	5	5	2
Rating	++++	+	+++	++	+	+	++++	+++	+++++

Keeping up to date with new trends
Statement rank order = tied rank 13.5. Rank total = 131.

	Sister Blue*	Red*	Gold	Green	Grey	Brown	White	Black	Pink
Rank order	16	13	20	17	11	16	3	24	11
Rating	+++	++	++	++	++	+	++++	+	+++

Disagreeing with a doctor's instructions for a patient
Statement rank order = tied rank 13.5. Rank total = 131.

	Sister Blue*	Red*	Gold	Green	Grey	Brown	White	Black	Pink
Rank order	23	2	13	6	22	10	17	17	21
Rating	+	+++++	+++	·++++	+	++	++	+	+

*not observed

Friction between staff
Statement rank order = 15. Rank total = 136.

	Sister Blue*	Red*	Gold	Green	Grey	Brown	White	Black	Pink
Rank order	25	11	25	11	18	22	6	9	9
Rating	+	+++	+	+++	+	+	+++	+++	+++

Doing things that are not part of my job
Statement rank order = 16. Rank total = 140.

	Sister Blue*	Red*	Gold	Green	Grey	Brown	White	Black	Pink
Rank order	22	19	19	20	12	4	2	23	19
Rating	+	+	++	++	+	+++++	+++++	+	++

Considering myself as manager
Statement rank order = tied rank 17.5. Rank total = 141.

	Sister Blue*	Red*	Gold	Green	Grey	Brown	White	Black	Pink
Rank order	17	21	24	7	17	19	8	21	7
Rating	++	+	+	++++	+	+	+++	+	++++

Getting the staff nurses to understand the sister's role
Statement rank order = tied rank 17.5. Rank total = 141

	Sister Blue*	Red*	Gold	Green	Grey	Brown	White	Black	Pink
Rank order	13	23	22	14	14	8	16	15	16
Rating	+++	+	+	+++	+	+++	++	++	++

Not having enough time to myself while on duty
Statement rank order = 19. Rank total = 145.

	Sister Blue*	Red*	Gold	Green	Grey	Brown	White	Black	Pink
Rank order	10	18	9	24	15	20	10	14	25
Rating	++++	+	+++	+	+	+	+++	++	+

*not observed

Finding someone to turn to when I need help
Statement rank order = 20. Rank total = 146.

	Sister Blue*	Red*	Gold	Green	Grey	Brown	White	Black	Pink
Rank order	20	24	15	12	9	9	23	19	15
Rating	++	+	+++	++	++	++	+	+	++

Making changes in the ward
Statement rank order = 21. Rank total = 154.

	Sister Blue*	Red*	Gold	Green	Grey	Brown	White	Black	Pink
Rank order	18	17	21	22	10	15	13	20	18
Rating	++	++	++	+	++	+	++	+	++

Getting the doctors to listen to my point of view
Statement rank order = 22. Rank total = 155.

	Sister Blue*	Red*	Gold	Green	Grey	Brown	White	Black	Pink
Rank order	21	12	14	10	19	17	22	18	22
Rating	+	+++	++	+++	+	+	+	+	+

Feeling isolated from other ward sisters
Statement rank order = 23. Rank total = 170.

	Sister Blue*	Red*	Gold	Green	Grey	Brown	White	Black	Pink
Rank order	19	10	16	25	24	25	11	16	24
Rating	++	+++	++	+	+	+	+++	++	+

Doing ward work in off-duty time
Statement rank order = 24. Rank total = 174.

	Sister Blue*	Red*	Gold	Green	Grey	Brown	White	Black	Pink
Rank order	15	22	11	23	21	24	25	10	23
Rating	+++	+	+++	+	+	+	+	+++	+

*not observed

Understanding my job responsibilities
Statement rank order = 25. Rank total = 181.

	Sister Blue*	Red*	Gold	Green	Grey	Brown	White	Black	Pink
Rank order	24	25	23	15	16	21	21	22	14
Rating	+	+	+	++	+	+	+	+	++

*not observed

Appendix 4

Ranking correlations

Spearman's rank order correlation coefficient
The following formula was used to find the relationship between pairs of rankings:

$$\rho = 1 - \frac{6 \, \Sigma \, D^2}{N(N^2 - 1)}$$

where D is the difference in ranks between the two sets of data and N is the number of items being ranked. Results fall between $+1$ (perfect positive correlation) and -1 (perfect negative correlation).

Correlation matrix

Sister	Blue	Red	Gold	Green	Grey	Brown	White	Black	Pink
Blue		0.48*	0.64*	0.38	0.59*	0.49*	0.02	0.62*	0.37
Red			0.36	0.31	0.19	0.37	0.12	0.38	0.24
Gold				0.29	0.14	0.32	−0.007	0.56*	0.21
Green					0.36	0.63*	−0.06	0.34	0.38
Grey						0.54*	−0.14	0.07	0.2
Brown							0.19	0.3	0.1
White								0.2	0.18
Black									0.17
Pink									

*P <0.01

Sample size	Significance level	
	0.05	0.01
25	0.336	0.475

Index